DIABETES

Simeon Margolis, M.D., Ph.D.

and

Christopher D. Saudek, M.D.

2002

DIABETES

Over the past decade, it has become increasingly clear that effective management of diabetes in the early stages of the disease has significant long-term benefits. Now, more than ever, people with diabetes have at their disposal effective ways to monitor their condition and numerous treatments to control their blood glucose. This year's White Paper reviews how diabetes produces symptoms and complications, explains the latest research and practice regarding the benefits of diet and lifestyle changes, and describes the newest advances in the treatment of the disease.

▪ ▪ ▪

Highlights:

▪ ▪ ▪

www.HopkinsAfter50.com
Visit us for the latest news on diabetes and other information that will complement your Johns Hopkins White Paper.

THE AUTHORS

Simeon Margolis, M.D., Ph.D., received his B.A., M.D., and Ph.D. from the Johns Hopkins University School of Medicine and performed his internship and residency at Johns Hopkins Hospital. He is currently a professor of medicine and biological chemistry at the Johns Hopkins University School of Medicine and medical editor of *The Johns Hopkins Medical Letter, Health After 50.* He has served on various committees for the Department of Health, Education and Welfare, including the National Diabetes Advisory Board and the Arteriosclerosis Specialized Centers of Research Review Committees. In addition, he has acted as a member of the Endocrinology and Metabolism Panel of the U.S. Food and Drug Administration.

A former weekly columnist for the *Baltimore Sun,* Dr. Margolis lectures regularly to medical students, physicians, and the general public on a wide variety of topics, such as the prevention of coronary heart disease, controlling cholesterol levels, the treatment of diabetes, and alternative medicine.

■ ■ ■

Christopher D. Saudek, M.D., received his B.A. from Harvard University and his M.D. from Cornell University Medical College. He trained in internal medicine at Chicago's Presbyterian-St. Luke's Hospital and in metabolism at Boston City Hospital and Harvard Medical School. After serving on the faculty at Cornell and winning a Robert Wood Johnson Health Policy Fellowship, Dr. Saudek joined the faculty of the Johns Hopkins University School of Medicine, where he is currently a professor of medicine, director of the Johns Hopkins Diabetes Center, and director of the General Clinical Research Center.

Currently president of the American Diabetes Association, Dr. Saudek is active in diabetes education and public health policy. His research focuses on the development of an implantable insulin pump, a topic on which he has published widely. He is author of *The Johns Hopkins Guide to Diabetes: For Today and Tomorrow.* In 1991, he was named Outstanding Clinician in Diabetes by the American Diabetes Association.

CONTENTS

DIABETES

Diabetes mellitus is a metabolic disorder characterized by abnormally high levels of blood glucose (sugar) due to the body's inadequate production of or insufficient response to insulin. Insulin is the hormone that controls the manufacture of glucose by the liver and allows muscle cells to remove glucose from the blood.

The disease is aptly named ("diabetes mellitus" is derived from the Greek word for siphon and the Latin word *mellitus,* meaning honey-sweet), since the passage of large amounts of sugar-laden urine is a key symptom of poorly controlled diabetes. The two principal dangers for people with diabetes are the immediate complications of high blood glucose levels and the long-term complications affecting the eyes, nerves, kidneys, and large blood vessels.

PREVALENCE OF DIABETES

In the United States, the prevalence of diabetes currently stands at about 15.7 million people, about a third of whom do not yet know they have the disease. A large portion, some 3.2 million, are age 65 or older. Since 1958, the number of people diagnosed with diabetes has more than tripled, rising from less than 1% of Americans to about 7% today. In 1999, an estimated 798,000 new cases of diabetes were diagnosed.

The direct medical costs of diabetes in the United States reached $44 billion in 1997, the most recent year for which such figures are available. Indirect costs—incurred from such factors as disability, work loss, and premature mortality—were estimated at $54 billion for the same period.

DIABETES TYPES

Diabetes is divided into two types. Type 1 diabetes usually emerges before age 30 and tends to come on suddenly. Type 2 diabetes, which accounts for 90% to 95% of diabetes cases, usually starts later in life. The onset tends to be more gradual, and blood glucose levels are more stable. Most patients with type 2 disease are obese.

Type 1 diabetes was once named insulin-dependent or juvenile diabetes, while type 2 diabetes was formerly called non-insulin dependent or adult diabetes. These terms are no longer used because some people with type 2 diabetes eventually require insulin, and be-

Insulin Defects in Type 1 and Type 2 Diabetes

After a meal, carbohydrates from food are converted to glucose (sugar) and enter the bloodstream. In response to the rise in blood glucose levels, the pancreas—a small, elongated gland located below and behind the stomach—produces the hormone insulin and secretes it into the bloodstream. Insulin allows glucose to enter cells, where it is used for energy or converted to a storage form for future use. Insulin also inhibits the release of glucose by the liver.

Insulin works similarly to a key in a lock. Specifically, insulin interacts with structures (called receptors) on the surface of cells to open small passageways through which glucose can enter cells. As a result, blood glucose levels fall and insulin production stops (see illustration A).

This process of moving glucose from the bloodstream into cells is disrupted in people with diabetes. In type 1 diabetes, damage to the pancreas by an abnormal autoimmune reaction reduces insulin production, so that little or no insulin is available to help get glucose into cells. The result is abnormally high levels of glucose in the blood, a condition called hyperglycemia (see illustration B). In type 2 diabetes, cells are less responsive to the actions of insulin. In other words, insulin interacts with the structures on the cell surfaces but has difficulty opening the small passageways, and insufficient glucose enters the cells. The pancreas compensates by producing more insulin, but over time it cannot produce enough to overcome the cells' reduced response. As in type 1 diabetes, the result is hyperglycemia (see illustration C). In addition, as type 2 diabetes progresses, the ability of the pancreas to produce insulin may also become impaired, making it even more difficult to remove glucose from the bloodstream.

A. Person Without Diabetes

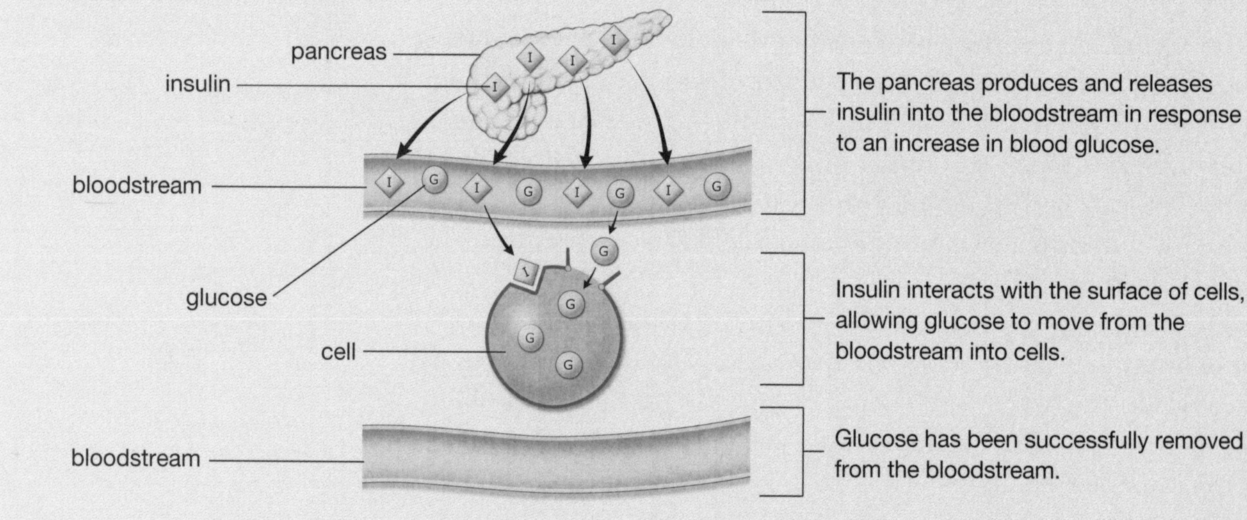
pancreas
insulin
bloodstream
glucose
cell
bloodstream
I
G
The pancreas produces and releases insulin into the bloodstream in response to an increase in blood glucose.
Insulin interacts with the surface of cells, allowing glucose to move from the bloodstream into cells.
Glucose has been successfully removed from the bloodstream.

cause there is a growing epidemic of type 2 disease in children.

IMPAIRED GLUCOSE TOLERANCE

In addition to diabetes, about 11% of American adults have impaired glucose tolerance, defined by abnormalities on a glucose tolerance test (blood glucose levels between 140 and 199 mg/dL two hours after ingesting 75 g of glucose). About 7% of these people go on to develop full-blown diabetes every year; many continue to manifest impaired glucose tolerance; and others return to nor-

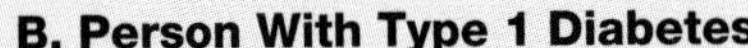

B. Person With Type 1 Diabetes

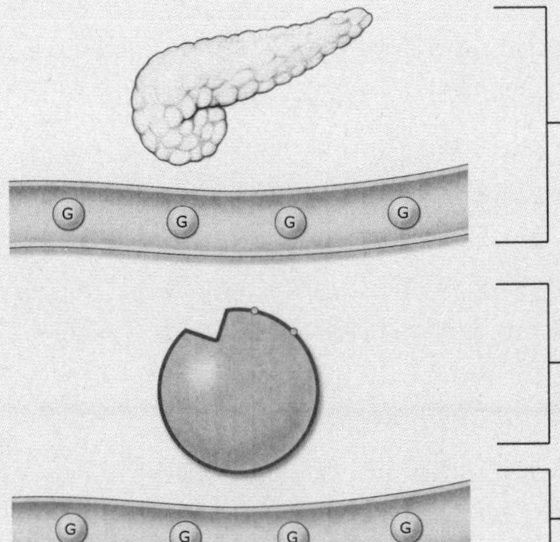

The pancreas produces and releases little or no insulin into the bloodstream in response to an increase in blood glucose.

Little or no insulin is available to interact with the surface of cells. Thus, glucose cannot enter cells.

Glucose remains in the bloodstream.

C. Person With Type 2 Diabetes

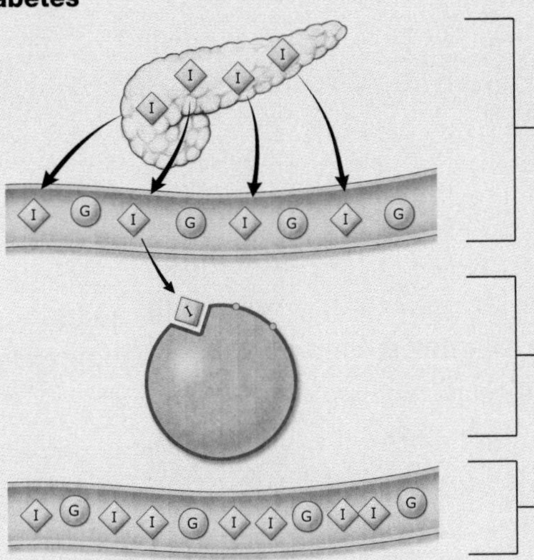

As in the person without diabetes, the pancreas produces and releases insulin into the bloodstream in response to an increase in blood glucose.

Insulin interacts with the surface of cells but has difficulty opening the passageways, preventing sufficient glucose from entering cells.

Glucose remains in the bloodstream. The pancreas responds by producing and releasing more insulin into the bloodstream.

mal without treatment. Individuals with impaired glucose tolerance are usually overweight and relatively resistant (less responsive) to the actions of insulin; often they also have high blood insulin levels (hyperinsulinemia).

Impaired glucose tolerance and hyperinsulinemia are associated with an increased risk of coronary heart disease (CHD). Individuals with impaired glucose tolerance should attain a healthy body weight, check for signs of diabetes, and try to modify other risk factors for CHD (such as cigarette smoking, high blood pressure, and elevated cholesterol levels).

CAUSES OF DIABETES

As mentioned before, diabetes is caused by an abnormality in the way the body uses glucose. This abnormality is due to insufficient production of insulin by the pancreas, resistance of the body's tissues to insulin action, or both.

Each cell needs a regular supply of glucose, which enters the blood from dietary carbohydrates or from the liver, where it is produced. When the right amount of insulin is present in the bloodstream, the liver shuts down its production of glucose. Glucose in the blood can then enter cells where it is used immediately for fuel. Some additional glucose is converted to glycogen in the liver and muscles and is stored there for future use. The body's ability to store glycogen is limited, however. Glucose not used immediately for energy or stored as glycogen is converted to triglycerides and stored in adipose (fatty) tissue.

Insulin—a hormone produced by cells in the parts of the pancreas known as islets of Langerhans—is the key regulator of glucose uptake by muscle and fat. As blood glucose levels rise after a meal, the pancreas responds by producing insulin. Insulin attaches to receptor sites on the surface of cells throughout the body. By a complex series of events within the cell, the binding of insulin to these receptors causes carrier proteins, called glucose transport proteins (GTPs), to move from inside the cell to the surface. Like little dump trucks, GTPs deliver glucose from outside the cell to the inside. But without the initial binding of insulin to cells, glucose cannot enter.

Another important function of insulin is to halt an excessive release of glucose from the liver into the bloodstream between meals. Special cells (also located in the islets of Langerhans) continuously monitor blood glucose levels and release insulin and glucagon, respectively, as needed. (Glucagon is a hormone that raises blood glucose levels by signaling the liver to convert amino acids and glycogen to glucose and to send the glucose into the bloodstream.) In diabetes, the balance between insulin and glucagon is thrown off by insufficient insulin production or by insulin resistance; the result is elevated blood glucose levels.

Type 1 diabetes is an autoimmune disease: The body produces antibodies that attack and damage the pancreatic cells, called beta cells, that secrete insulin. At first, the ability of the beta cells to secrete insulin is merely impaired, but eventually (usually in less than a year) they produce little or no insulin. Fortunately, body tissues respond normally to insulin delivered by injection, and so people with type 1 diabetes can compensate by injecting insulin regularly. Although heredity plays some role in type 1 diabetes, most patients have no known family history of diabetes.

Resistance to the action of insulin is common in obesity and is a uniform feature of type 2 diabetes. In this disorder, the body's tissues (primarily the liver and muscles) become less sensitive to insulin action. In order for cells to get the glucose they need, the pancreas must increase its production of insulin. Diabetes results when the pancreas is unable to secrete enough extra insulin to overcome the tissue resistance. The majority of patients with type 2 diabetes can be treated with lifestyle measures (diet and exercise) or oral drugs, but about 40% need insulin injections to achieve adequate control of their blood glucose.

Heredity plays an important role in type 2 diabetes. In a study of 218 type 2 patients (age 35 to 74), 66% reported at least one relative with diabetes and 46% had at least two relatives with the disorder. In particular, patients whose mother had diabetes were two times more likely to get the disease than those whose father had it—33% vs. 17%, respectively. Of the women with diabetes, 11% had at least one child with diabetes, whereas only 4% of the men with diabetes had a child with the disorder.

People can also develop diabetes because of some other disorder. For example, diabetes can result from diseases that destroy the pancreas—such as hemochromatosis (an excessive absorption and storage of iron) or chronic pancreatitis (inflammation of the pancreas)—or from surgical removal of the pancreas, such as for cancer. Tumors of certain endocrine organs can cause diabetes due to overproduction of hormones that interfere with insulin action. For example, the growth hormone produced by some tumors of the pituitary gland, cortisol or epinephrine from adrenal tumors, and glucagon from pancreatic tumors can all raise blood glucose levels. Corticosteroids, used to treat asthma or arthritis, or the cholesterol-lowering agent niacin, for example, may also bring out latent diabetes.

PREVENTION OF DIABETES

Prevention of diabetes is, of course, preferable to its treatment. One study, the Diabetes Prevention Trial—Type 1, is underway to see if type 1 diabetes can be avoided by use of insulin injections or insulin capsules in people at increased risk for type 1 diabetes. In other research, immunosuppressive drugs to prevent type 1 dia-

NEW RESEARCH

Cigarette Smoking Linked To Increased Diabetes Risk

Cigarette smoking is a known risk factor for cardiovascular disease. A new study now shows that smoking is also related to an increased risk of type 2 diabetes.

To evaluate the relationship between smoking and diabetes, researchers observed 21,068 U.S. male physicians, age 40 to 84, for an average of 12 years. During this time, 770 of the men developed type 2 diabetes.

The researchers found that the number of cigarettes the physicians smoked at the beginning of the study was strongly associated with their risk of developing diabetes. Those who smoked 20 or more cigarettes a day were 70% more likely to develop diabetes than those who had never smoked; among those who smoked fewer than 20 cigarettes a day, the risk was increased by 50%. Former smokers, however, had a risk similar to those who had never smoked.

The risk of type 2 diabetes associated with smoking is similar to that associated with mild obesity or high blood pressure, according to the study authors. They estimate that about 10% of cases of type 2 diabetes result from cigarette smoking.

THE AMERICAN JOURNAL OF MEDICINE
Volume 109, page 538
November 2000

betes have yet to produce encouraging results.

One of the immunosuppressive drugs, cyclosporine, reduced the need for insulin in some people when started during the first two months after the onset of type 1 diabetes. This effect, however, depended on the continued administration of cyclosporine; relapse, with the need to restart insulin, occurred promptly after the drug was stopped. Unfortunately, long-term use of cyclosporine is associated with kidney damage. Therefore, neither cyclosporine nor any other immunosuppressive drug is currently considered an acceptable approach to the prevention or treatment of type 1 diabetes.

Efforts to prevent type 2 diabetes are especially important for individuals at highest risk for developing the disease—those who have impaired glucose tolerance, are overweight, have a family history of the disorder, belong to a high-risk ethnic group (such as blacks, Hispanics, or Native Americans), or have a history of diabetes during pregnancy (gestational diabetes).

The Diabetes Prevention Program recently showed that the drug metformin (Glucophage) is effective in reducing the risk of developing diabetes in patients at high risk, and that diet and exercise are even more effective. (See the sidebar on page 29.)

In addition, a high-fiber diet may decrease the risk of developing type 2 diabetes. A 2000 study of 35,988 women found that women who consumed the most fiber from cereal had a 36% reduced risk of developing type 2 diabetes compared with those consuming the least.

ACUTE SYMPTOMS OF DIABETES

The initial symptoms of diabetes are usually related to hyperglycemia, the medical term for high blood glucose. The onset of type 1 diabetes is often sudden, and diabetic ketoacidosis (see page 8) may be the first indication of the disease. In contrast, type 2 diabetes may develop so gradually that some patients notice few or no symptoms for a number of years. They may initially complain of symptoms from chronic complications, such as peripheral neuropathy (nerve damage in the hands or feet). In other cases, the diagnosis of type 2 diabetes is made by a routine laboratory test in patients who are symptom-free.

Classic presenting symptoms. The classic presenting symptoms of diabetes are an increased frequency of urination (polyuria), increased thirst and fluid intake (polydipsia), and, as the disease pro-

On the Rise: Obesity and Type 2 Diabetes

Obesity is a major contributing factor to type 2 diabetes. Research indicates that as a person's weight increases, the risk of type 2 diabetes also increases.

The prevalence of both obesity and diabetes has increased rapidly in recent years (see the graph below), and many knowledgeable observers now consider these problems to be "epidemics." Between 1991 and 1999, the percentage of the U.S. population diagnosed with diabetes increased by 38%—from 5.0% to 6.9% of the population. (And most studies indicate that almost a third of people with diabetes have not been diagnosed.) Over that same period, the percentage of people classified as obese rose by 57%—from 12.0% to 18.9% of the population.

Unless efforts are made to limit these increases, researchers suspect that these trends will continue.

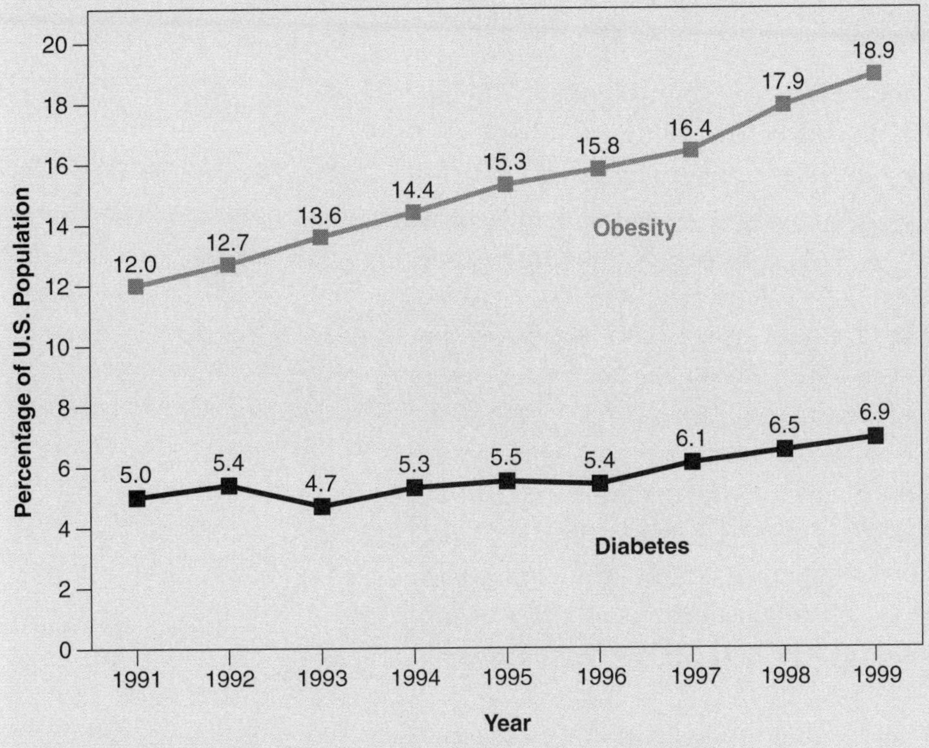

A common way of measuring obesity is body mass index (BMI), a measure of weight in relation to height. To calculate your BMI, multiply your weight (in pounds) by 704. Then multiply your height (in inches) by itself. Your BMI is the first number divided by the second. People with a BMI of 30 or greater are considered obese, while those with a BMI between 25 and 29.9 are considered overweight.

Source: Centers for Disease Control and Prevention.

gresses, weight loss despite increased hunger and food intake (polyphagia). These symptoms, all caused by high blood glucose and the accompanying "spillover" of excess glucose into the urine, can be prevented by maintaining reasonable blood glucose levels. Other common symptoms include blurred vision due to changing levels of glucose in the eye; weakness and fatigue; recurrent vaginal yeast infections; and skin infections. These symptoms are transient, do not indicate any permanent damage, and can be eliminated by achieving control of blood glucose levels.

When people who are receiving treatment for diabetes experience these symptoms, they should adjust their therapy. Those with type 2 diabetes who are using exercise and diet alone to control blood glucose levels may need to start taking oral medications or insulin. People already taking insulin might have to adjust the dosage after consulting their health care professional. In either case, it is important for individuals to drink plenty of water and make sure they are correctly following their prescribed treatment plan (for example, maintaining regular eating habits).

Diabetic ketoacidosis. This acute complication of diabetes results when a nearly complete lack of insulin forces the body to utilize energy from sources other than glucose—namely, acids released from fat tissue stores. These fatty acids are broken down by the liver into several strong acids known as ketone bodies. The accumulation of ketone bodies increases the acidity of the blood (metabolic acidosis) to dangerous levels.

In addition, elevated blood glucose (due to the lack of insulin action) leads to the excretion of large amounts of glucose and water in the urine, causing severe dehydration. Diabetic ketoacidosis is generally limited to patients who have type 1 diabetes, but it can occasionally occur when those with type 2 diabetes are under physical stress, such as during an infection.

Symptoms of ketoacidosis include fruity breath; nausea and vomiting; slow, deep respiration; changes in mental status (initial confusion can deepen into coma); and—finally—collapse of the cardiovascular system. Diabetic ketoacidosis is a medical emergency that usually requires immediate hospitalization. Death can occur, but the vast majority of patients recover with aggressive administration of insulin and fluids.

Hyperosmolar nonketotic states. The stress of an injury or a major illness, such as a stroke, heart attack, or severe infection, can raise blood glucose to extremely high levels in type 2 patients. While their insulin concentrations are adequate to avert excessive ketone body production, they cannot prevent high blood glucose levels and the rise in blood osmolarity ("thickening" of the blood) that gives this condition its name. Severe dehydration worsens the problem, and patients develop lethargy, prostration, confusion, and, in extreme cases, coma.

In about a third of patients with this condition, it is the first indication of their diabetes. Like ketoacidosis, hyperosmolar states can be fatal if not rapidly treated with insulin and large amounts of fluids. Patients experiencing the above-mentioned symptoms should contact their doctor. If unconsciousness occurs, an ambulance should be called immediately.

DIAGNOSIS AND OFFICE FOLLOW-UP OF DIABETES

Symptoms may suggest the presence of diabetes, but laboratory tests are needed to make a definitive diagnosis. In an effort to promote the early detection of diabetes, and thus help reduce the risk of its complications, the American Diabetes Association (ADA) recommends that individuals age 45 and older be tested every three years.

The presence of certain factors that heighten the risk for developing diabetes should prompt earlier and more frequent testing. These factors are obesity; having a first-degree relative (parent or sibling) with diabetes; being in a high-risk ethnic group (including black, Hispanic, and Native American); delivering a baby weighing more than 9 lbs or being diagnosed with gestational diabetes; high blood pressure (140/90 mm Hg or higher, also called hypertension); low HDL cholesterol levels (less than 40 mg/dL); high triglycerides (200 mg/dL or higher); and impaired glucose tolerance. If diabetes is diagnosed, the progress of the disease is monitored through regular physical examinations and laboratory tests.

Laboratory Tests

Diabetes is diagnosed by measuring blood glucose levels. The diagnosis is made when a blood glucose level greater than 200 mg/dL in any blood sample is associated with the classic symptoms of high blood glucose—thirst, frequent urination, and weight loss. A diagnosis of diabetes is also made when a fasting blood glucose level is above 125 mg/dL on at least two tests. Fasting blood glucose values between 110 and 125 mg/dL define impaired fasting glucose and identify patients who should be followed more closely. A normal fasting blood glucose level is less than 110 mg/dL.

Oral glucose tolerance test. An oral glucose tolerance test may also be used to diagnose diabetes, but it is not necessary when either of the above criteria for diabetes is satisfied. In this test, an individual ingests a drink containing 75 g of glucose. The diagnosis of diabetes is made if two hours later the blood glucose level is 200 mg/dL or more. Impaired glucose tolerance is defined by two-hour glucose levels between 140 and 200 mg/dL. Glucose levels of 140 mg/dL and below at two hours are normal.

Hemoglobin A1c test. A test for hemoglobin A1c (HbA1c), also known as glycohemoglobin or glycated hemoglobin, is used to assess blood glucose control over the previous two to three months in people already diagnosed with diabetes. The test measures the amount of glucose attached to hemoglobin (the oxygen-carrying

NEW RESEARCH

Timing of Blood Test May Affect Accuracy of Diabetes Diagnosis

A fasting blood glucose test is commonly used to diagnose diabetes. But when the test is performed in the afternoon—rather than the morning—the likelihood of missing diabetes may be increased, a new study finds.

Researchers measured fasting blood glucose levels in 12,882 people (age 20 and older) with no previous diagnosis of diabetes. About half of the people received the blood test in the morning; the other half in the afternoon.

Fasting blood glucose levels were significantly lower in people given the test in the afternoon than in the morning (92.4 mg/dL vs. 97.4 mg/dL). As a result, half as many patients met the criteria for diabetes in the afternoon group as in the morning group (1.4% vs. 2.8%).

The current standard for diagnosing diabetes is a fasting blood glucose of 126 mg/dL or more. Because the standard is based on blood glucose levels measured in the morning, and blood glucose tends to be higher at that time, the study authors note that some people with diabetes could be missed if tested in the afternoon. They also note that physicians should repeat the test on a different day to confirm the diagnosis, regardless of whether the test is given in the morning or afternoon.

JOURNAL OF THE AMERICAN MEDICAL ASSOCIATION
Volume 284, page 3157
December 27, 2000

protein in red blood cells that gives blood its color). This amount increases as the blood glucose level rises. Since hemoglobin circulates in the blood until the red blood cells die (half the red blood cells are replaced every 12 to 16 weeks), the hemoglobin A1c test is a useful tool for measuring average blood glucose levels over time. (For more information on the hemoglobin A1c test, see the feature on the opposite page.)

A similar test, called the fructosamine test, also measures glucose bound to protein. The results reflect average blood glucose levels over the preceding two weeks.

Other tests. In addition to measures of blood glucose and hemoglobin A1c or fructosamine, initial and subsequent evaluations may also include tests of blood urea nitrogen (BUN), blood creatinine, and protein (albumin) in the urine to evaluate possible kidney damage, as well as measurements of triglycerides and total, LDL, and HDL cholesterol to assess risk factors for CHD.

Medical History and Physical Examination

Certain features of the patient's medical history and physical examination are particularly important in people with diabetes. The history should cover time and circumstances of the diagnosis; dietary habits; weight history; use of oral blood glucose-lowering drugs; insulin use, including amounts and time of administration; symptoms of long-term diabetic complications; effectiveness of blood glucose control (symptoms of high blood glucose and blood glucose values); frequency and timing of symptoms of hypoglycemia (low blood glucose); history of diabetic ketoacidosis; alcohol and tobacco use; exercise habits; family history of diabetes, CHD, and stroke; and other medications taken.

A physical examination should emphasize weight; blood pressure; examination of the eyes with dilated pupils (by an ophthalmologist, a medical doctor who specializes in diseases of the eye); inspection of the feet for pulses, infection, cuts, blisters, or calluses; and neurological testing for reflexes and loss of sensation.

LONG-TERM COMPLICATIONS OF DIABETES

Chronic, or long-term, complications can occur in both types of diabetes and in many cases are directly related to elevated blood glucose levels. Long-term complications include microvascular disease (abnormalities of small blood vessels), neuropathy (nerve damage), changes to the skin, gums, and teeth, and macrovascular disease

Hemoglobin A1c Testing and Diabetes

Monitoring blood glucose levels and maintaining tight glucose control are essential elements in the management of both type 1 and type 2 diabetes. Although self-monitoring of blood glucose is an important part of management, it can only reveal a person's glucose levels at the moment when the blood is drawn. To monitor average blood glucose levels over a two- to three-month period, doctors use another blood test, called hemoglobin A1c (HbA1c). Knowing your average blood glucose levels over time tells you if your diabetes is under control, how well your treatments are working, and what your chances are of developing certain complications from diabetes.

What Is Hemoglobin A1c?
After a meal, glucose is absorbed from the intestine and circulates in the blood. It is also made in the liver and released into the blood between meals. The body's cells take up most of the glucose from the blood. This glucose is used at once as an energy source, or is stored for later use as fat or as glycogen in the liver. Some of the glucose attaches to hemoglobin, a protein found in red blood cells that carries oxygen throughout the body and gives blood its red color.

Glucose remains combined with hemoglobin for the life of a red blood cell—about 120 days. The combination of glucose and hemoglobin is called glycosylated hemoglobin, glycohemoglobin, or glycated hemoglobin. Its main component is HbA1c. When glucose levels on average are high, the amount of HbA1c increases. Because glycosylated hemoglobin stays in the blood for many weeks, measuring its levels gives a picture of average blood glucose control over the previous two to three months.

What Do the Test Results Mean?
In healthy people without diabetes, HbA1c levels are typically between 4% and 6%. The American Diabetes Association (ADA) recommends that people with diabetes aim to reduce their HbA1c levels to below 7%, a level that indicates good blood glucose control. If a person with diabetes has HbA1c values exceeding 8%, the ADA suggests that the patient and doctor take action to lower these levels.

Elevated levels of HbA1c increase the risk of experiencing diabetes-related complications such as eye, kidney, and nerve damage. Results from the Diabetes Control and Complications Trial and the United Kingdom Prospective Diabetes Study show that people with type 1 and type 2 diabetes who lower their HbA1c levels to near 7% can significantly delay or prevent the onset of complications.

How Often Should You Be Tested?
The ADA recommends HbA1c testing twice a year for people with diabetes whose levels of HbA1c are stable. They suggest testing every three months for people with diabetes whose treatment plan has changed or whose HbA1c levels are greater than 8%.

Only about half of people with diabetes have received a test for HbA1c. So if you do not know what your levels are, be sure that your doctor performs the test. Your test results will tell you how well your diabetes is controlled and how close you are to your target level. Because labs can use various techniques to measure HbA1c levels, try to have the analysis done at the same lab each time.

(abnormalities of large blood vessels). They typically appear only after years or decades of the disease, and their development is *not* inevitable.

There is definitive evidence that good control of blood glucose and control of other risk factors, such as high blood pressure, can eliminate or postpone diabetic complications, and may reduce their severity if they do occur. However, improved glucose control may not reverse these complications once they appear. Treatments for long-term complications of diabetes are covered on pages 47–56.

Microvascular Disease

Microvascular disease due to diabetes affects the eyes and kidneys.

Retinopathy. Diabetic retinopathy, the most common diabetic eye complication and the leading cause of blindness among U.S. adults, is damage to the retina (the light-sensitive nerve tissue at the back of the eye that transmits visual images to the brain). This damage is caused by changes in the tiny blood vessels that supply the retina.

In the early stages of retinopathy—called nonproliferative retinopathy—the retinal vessels weaken and develop bulges (microaneurysms) that may leak blood (hemorrhage) or fluid (exudate) into the surrounding tissue. Vision is rarely affected during this stage of retinopathy, but annual eye examinations should be performed by an ophthalmologist to ensure that the condition does not progress. Later on, however, patients can develop proliferative retinopathy, when fragile new blood vessels begin to grow on the retina and into the vitreous humor (the jelly-like substance inside the back of the eye). These abnormal vessels are prone to rupture and bleed into the vitreous humor, causing blurred vision or temporary blindness. If detected early enough, proliferative retinopathy can be treated with laser surgery (see pages 47–48). (For more information on the stages of diabetic retinopathy, see the feature on pages 18–19.)

The Diabetes Control and Complications Trial (DCCT) and the United Kingdom Prospective Diabetes Study (UKPDS) showed that maintaining lower blood glucose levels in people with type 1 and type 2 diabetes, respectively, can significantly reduce the risk of developing retinopathy or slow its progression (see pages 22–24). In another large study, people with the highest hemoglobin A1c levels at the start of the study had nearly a three times greater risk of developing retinopathy after 10 years than those with the lowest levels. Among patients taking insulin, those with the highest hemoglobin A1c levels had a 90% greater risk of developing retinopathy than those with the lowest levels. Risk of progression of existing retinopathy was also increased in patients with the highest hemoglobin A1c levels. The researchers concluded that lowering blood glucose levels significantly reduces both the incidence and progression of retinopathy. The UKPDS also showed that even modest reductions in blood pressure were associated with a marked reduction in retinopathy.

About half of those with untreated proliferative retinopathy will become blind within five years, compared to just 5% of those who receive laser treatment. Regular eye exams offer the best chance of detecting retinopathy in its treatable stages. Nevertheless, only half of all people with diagnosed diabetes in the United States have a yearly eye examination by an ophthalmologist. People with type 1 diabetes should have a dilated eye exam every year, starting five years after diabetes is diagnosed; those with type 2 diabetes should have one at diagnosis and annually after that. People with both type 2 diabetes and high blood pressure should be particularly vigilant about having eye exams, since one study found that retinopathy develops earlier and is more severe in those with a systolic blood pressure (the upper number in a blood pressure reading) above 140 mm Hg.

Nephropathy. About 30% to 40% of people with type 1 diabetes and 20% of those with type 2 diabetes develop nephropathy (kidney damage) that can lead to kidney failure. The rate of nephropathy is decreasing, however, due to wide recognition of the benefits of better diabetic control shown in the DCCT. The DCCT showed that intensive diabetes management could reduce kidney damage by 50%. For more information about preserving kidney function, see the feature on pages 50–51.

Neuropathy

About 60% to 70% of people with diabetes develop some form of nerve damage (neuropathy), though they may experience no symptoms. Neuropathy typically develops slowly. The best way to prevent it is to maintain good control of blood glucose. According to the DCCT, tight control can decrease the risk of neuropathy by 60%.

Diabetes can cause three types of neuropathy: peripheral neuropathy, mononeuropathy, and autonomic neuropathy. Most common is peripheral neuropathy, a slow, progressive loss of function of the sensory nerves in the limbs that causes numbness, tingling, and pain in the legs and hands on both sides of the body.

Mononeuropathy, which results from disruption of the blood supply to one or more nerves, leads to the sudden onset of pain or weakness in the area of the body served by the affected nerve. Mononeuropathy is apparently caused by blockages in flow through small arteries supplying blood to a nerve, similar to a mini-stroke. While the symptoms of mononeuropathy gradually improve over two to six months without any treatment, nerve damage due to peripheral neuropathy responds to diabetic control slowly, if at all.

Autonomic neuropathy damages nerves to the digestive tract, bladder, heart, and other internal organs. For more on autonomic neuropathy, see the feature on pages 14–15.

Glaucoma and Cataracts

These treatable eye conditions occur with increased frequency in people with diabetes. There is some evidence that elevated levels of

NEW RESEARCH

Older Women With Diabetes May Have Increased Fracture Risk

Diabetes is not usually considered a risk factor for osteoporosis (bone loss that makes the bones more fragile), but a new study shows that diabetes may contribute to a higher risk of bone fractures in older women.

In this study of 9,654 women, age 65 or older, 657 women had type 2 diabetes. Researchers measured the women's bone mineral density (BMD) at baseline and then determined the number of fractures that occurred over an average of nine years.

Women with diabetes had a higher BMD than the nondiabetic group, but surprisingly they also had a higher risk of certain types of fractures. Participants on insulin had the highest risk of foot and ankle fractures, though the risk of spinal fractures was not increased in any of the participants with diabetes.

There are several possible explanations for the discrepancy between BMD and fracture risk. First, BMD tests focus on bones in the spine, hip, and forearm, instead of those of the foot and ankle, which are apparently prone to fracture in diabetic people. Also, impaired blood flow may affect the rate of bone turnover and make fractures more likely even though BMD is high. In addition, increased falls due to diabetic neuropathy or poor vision may explain the higher fracture risk.

THE JOURNAL OF CLINICAL ENDOCRINOLOGY & METABOLISM
Volume 86, pages 29 and 32
March 2001

Diabetic Autonomic Neuropathy

About 60% to 70% of people with diabetes develop nerve damage, a condition called diabetic neuropathy. Most common is peripheral neuropathy, which is characterized by pain or numbness in the feet and hands. But diabetes can also damage the nerves that control the body's internal organs, resulting in autonomic neuropathy. Autonomic neuropathy affects up to 30% of people with diabetes. Maintaining good blood glucose control is the best way to prevent autonomic neuropathy in addition to other types of diabetic neuropathy.

What Is Autonomic Neuropathy?
A complex network of nerves carries messages back and forth between the brain and the rest of the body. These messages are needed for the body to function properly. Autonomic neuropathy occurs when the autonomic nerves in this network become damaged. Autonomic nerves regulate bodily functions that are not under voluntary control, such as digestion, heart rate, and blood pressure. These functions are impaired by injury to the autonomic nerves.

Researchers are not sure what causes autonomic neuropathy in people with diabetes, but they suspect that high blood glucose is an important factor. Excess blood glucose may impair the ability of autonomic nerves to transmit messages by damaging the nerve or the blood vessels that provide nutrients and oxygen to the nerve.

Who Is at Risk?
Autonomic neuropathy most often occurs in people who have had diabetes for many years and who have had problems controlling their blood glucose levels. Men are at greater risk than women, and so are smokers, heavy drinkers, and people over age 40. Most people with autonomic neuropathy also have significant peripheral neuropathy.

The best way to prevent autonomic neuropathy, or at least to delay its onset, is to keep blood glucose levels as close to normal as possible. Research also shows that exercising regularly, eating a healthy diet, quitting smoking, and limiting alcohol are also important for prevention.

What Are the Symptoms?
The symptoms of autonomic neuropathy vary from person to person and depend upon what organs are affected by the nerve damage. In some people, neuropathy affects many parts of the body, while in others the damage is limited to a single organ. The inset box at right shows the parts of the body that are most likely to be affected by autonomic neuropathy and the symptoms that typically result.

If you develop any of the symptoms listed in the table, be sure to tell your doctor. Because many of the symptoms can have causes other than nerve damage, your doctor will ask questions about the symptoms and perform a physical exam. Tests to measure the function of the autonomic nerves may also be needed.

How Is It Treated?
The most important step in treating autonomic neuropathy is to make sure your blood glucose levels are under control. Doing so will help to slow the progression of neuropathy, and may even reverse the nerve damage in some cases. You should also quit smoking and reduce the amount of alcohol that you drink.

Efforts to develop drugs that can reverse nerve damage have not been successful. Treatments for the symptoms of autonomic neuropathy are available, however, and are summarized below.

• **Stomach problems.** The stomach problems associated with autonomic neuropathy, called gastroparesis, occur when nerve damage slows the emptying of the stomach after a meal. Symptoms of gastroparesis can often be improved by eating smaller, more frequent meals and avoiding foods that are high in fat and fiber. If this approach doesn't work, your doctor may prescribe the drug metoclopramide (Reglan). Some studies show that the antibiotic erythromycin may also be helpful.

• **Bowel problems.** To prevent alternating bouts of diarrhea and constipation, experts recommend eating

sorbitol, a sugar formed from glucose, within the lens of the eye enhance cataract formation in people with diabetes. While cataracts are usually treated only when they begin to interfere with vision, it is important to be tested regularly for glaucoma, since serious damage may occur before it causes symptoms.

Skin Changes

A violet-colored area of thinned skin, an inch or more in diameter, on the front of the lower part of the leg (necrobiosis lipoidica dia-

foods that are high in fiber (such as fruits, vegetables, and grains) and taking one to three tablespoons of psyllium (for example, Metamucil) each day. Diarrhea is usually treated with over-the-counter anti-diarrheal medications; constipation is relieved with cathartics such as prunes or laxatives. For difficult-to-treat diarrhea, antibiotics and other prescription medications may be necessary.

• **Bladder problems.** Difficulties emptying the bladder, which can increase the risk of bladder infections, can be minimized by applying pressure to the bladder while urinating or using a technique called "double voiding" that involves urinating a second time several minutes after the first. When bladder control is the problem, visiting the bathroom at regular intervals (for example, every two to three hours), rather than waiting until your bladder is full, may be helpful. If necessary, medications can be prescribed to deal with bladder problems.

• **Sexual dysfunction.** Erectile dysfunction is the most common symptom of autonomic neuropathy in men. Several treatment options are available. Least invasive is sildenafil (Viagra), an oral medication that has been shown to be effective in up to 50% of men with diabetes. This drug must be used with caution in men with heart disease, high blood pressure, or macular degeneration (an eye disease), and cannot be used at all by men taking nitrates for the treatment of angina. Other treatments for erectile dysfunction include drugs that are injected or inserted into the penis, and vacuum devices. In women, vaginal dryness during intercourse can be alleviated with the use of lubricants.

• **Dizziness.** Dizziness or lightheadedness upon rising, either from a sitting or reclining position, occurs in people with autonomic neuropathy because blood pools in the legs and causes a drop in blood pressure. One way to avoid this drop in blood pressure is to rise slowly. You can also try raising the head of your bed or ask your doctor about specially-designed elastic stockings that help blood return from your legs to your heart. If you do not have high blood pressure or heart problems, your doctor may recommend that you increase the amount of sodium in your diet or take a drug called fludrocortisone (Florinef) that helps the kidneys retain salt. Increasing the amount of sodium in your body raises blood volume, which helps to keep blood pressure from dropping when you rise.

• **Rapid or irregular heart beat.** Your doctor may prescribe medications to slow the heart and to prevent irregular heart beats.

• **Sweating.** Because there are no treatments for abnormal sweating, try to avoid situations in which you might become overheated.

Affected Part of the Body	Symptoms
Stomach	Heartburn, bloating, nausea and vomiting
Bowel	Alternating bouts of diarrhea and constipation
Bladder	Difficulty in emptying the bladder (urinary retention), difficulty controlling the bladder (urinary incontinence)
Sexual organs	Erectile dysfunction in men, vaginal dryness and decreased sexual response in women
Blood vessels	Dizziness or lightheadedness upon rising from a sitting or reclining position (orthostatic hypotension)
Heart	Rapid heart beat (90 beats or more at rest), irregular heart beat
Skin	Abnormal sweating (legs and arms sweat very little, while the central part of the body sweats excessively), excessive sweating while eating or at night

beticorum, or NLD) may occur occasionally in people with diabetes. At times, an ulcer (open sore) may appear in its center. Although no effective treatment is currently available for NLD, the condition only looks alarming and is not particularly harmful unless the affected skin becomes infected. (People with diabetes are, in general, more prone to skin infections.) Another characteristic skin change in diabetes is the shin spot, a darkly colored round lesion about half an inch in diameter. In addition, either a loss or an overgrowth of underlying fat tissue may occur at sites of insulin injection.

Dental Changes

Diabetes can lead to complications affecting the teeth and gums, and dry mouth is also common. Because saliva normally protects against bacterial growth in the mouth, and insufficient saliva permits dental plaque and food particles to accumulate, people with poorly controlled diabetes are more likely to develop cavities. As a result of excess plaque formation, two gum disorders, gingivitis and the more serious periodontitis, are also more common in people with diabetes. On the other hand, people who control their diabetes well may actually reduce their chance of cavities by selecting a diet that is lower in simple sugars (which can encourage cavity formation) and by following an oral health regimen carefully. Another dental complication, a burning sensation in the mouth and tongue, can result from dry mouth or diabetic neuropathy.

Macrovascular Disease

Diabetic patients are highly susceptible to the atherosclerotic narrowing of large blood vessels that causes such complications as heart attacks, strokes, and poor circulation to the legs (peripheral vascular disease).

Insulin resistance syndrome. Medical scientists and physicians have recognized a common constellation of findings—resistance to insulin; diabetes; abdominal obesity; high blood pressure; high triglyceride levels (hypertriglyceridemia) and low HDL cholesterol levels in the blood; and premature CHD—known as syndrome X, insulin resistance syndrome, or metabolic syndrome. A genetic predisposition to insulin resistance, as well as an accumulation of fat in the abdomen, may trigger the abnormalities of this syndrome. The liver releases too much glucose, the glucose cannot be used efficiently, and the pancreas increases its production of insulin to compensate. The result is elevated blood levels of insulin, which causes hypertriglyceridemia and low levels of HDL cholesterol. (One theory proposes that high blood levels of insulin may also lead to high blood pressure by reducing the excretion of sodium from the body. The additional sodium could cause a greater retention of water in the bloodstream, and the resulting rise in blood volume would raise blood pressure.) Blood glucose levels may gradually rise as insulin production by the pancreas can no longer keep up with the insulin resistance; impaired glucose tolerance and then diabetes often develop.

Together, these abnormalities raise the incidence of angina (episodes of chest pain owing to an inadequate supply of blood to the heart), heart attacks, strokes, and peripheral vascular disease. Long-term studies have shown that the higher the fasting blood insulin levels and the larger the amount of abdominal fat, the greater the likelihood of death from CHD. Although these risks occur even when blood glucose is only slightly elevated, they are magnified when patients become diabetic. The adverse consequences of insulin resistance syndrome can be avoided by controlling body weight (preferably through a combination of diet and exercise), blood pressure, and blood lipids (cholesterol and triglycerides).

Coronary heart disease. People with diabetes have a two to four times greater likelihood of having CHD, narrowing of the coronary arteries by atherosclerosis. The incidence of heart attacks is particularly increased in women with diabetes. One Finnish study of almost 1,300 people, age 65 to 74, found that 15% of those with type 2 diabetes had a heart attack over a period of 3½ years, compared with 3% of those without diabetes. The leading risk factors for people with diabetes in this study were elevated hemoglobin A1c levels and long duration of diabetes.

Other research has shown that diabetes decreases the normal tendency of the coronary arteries to widen—and thereby increase blood flow to the heart—during exercise. As a result, people with diabetes are at greater risk for angina and heart attacks. The Framingham Heart Study (an ongoing study in Massachusetts) and many others have shown that diabetes adds significantly to conventional risk factors like smoking, high blood pressure, and elevated LDL ("bad") or low HDL ("good") cholesterol levels. In fact, another Finnish study recently found that even when people with type 2 diabetes have no prior history of heart disease, they have the same risk of a heart attack as those without diabetes who have already had a heart attack. These data underscore the fact that people with diabetes should be especially attentive to *all* risk factors in guarding against CHD.

Stroke. In general, people with diabetes have twice the risk of stroke. According to a separate published analysis of the first Finnish study mentioned above (which followed nearly 1,300 people), women with diabetes had a two-times greater risk of stroke than those without diabetes. Men with diabetes had no overall increase in strokes, possibly due to the small number of strokes among the men in the study. High hemoglobin A1c levels, elevated blood glucose (following an overnight fast or two hours after glucose ingestion), and long duration of diabetes were important risk factors for stroke. The researchers conducting the study suspect that high

NEW RESEARCH

Diabetes Associated With Increased Calcium in the Coronary Arteries

A recent study shows that people with diabetes tend to have an increased buildup of calcium in the coronary arteries. Coronary artery calcium is a marker of atherosclerosis and a risk factor for coronary heart disease (CHD).

Investigators used electron beam computed tomography to measure the amount of calcium in the coronary arteries of 3,389 people (average age about 55), including 195 people with diabetes (mostly type 2).

Average coronary artery calcium scores were higher for people of all ages and both sexes with diabetes than in people without diabetes. Men tended to have higher calcium scores than women, and men older than age 69 with diabetes had the highest calcium scores of all the study groups.

The investigators write that preliminary evidence from other studies suggests that modifying CHD risk factors, such as improving cholesterol levels and quitting smoking, may slow the buildup of coronary artery calcium.

DIABETES RESEARCH AND CLINICAL PRACTICE
Volume 53, page 55
July 2001

Stages of Diabetic Retinopathy

Diabetic retinopathy is a long-term complication of diabetes marked by changes in the blood vessels in the retina, the light-sensitive nerve tissue at the back of the eye. When damaged, these vessels may leak blood and eventually develop fragile branches and scar tissue—changes that can blur or distort the visual images transmitted to the brain.

The prevalence of retinopathy is strongly related to how long a person has had diabetes. After 20 years, nearly all people with type 1 diabetes experience some degree of retinopathy, as do more than 60% of individuals with type 2 disease. Factors associated with the development of diabetic retinopathy include poor blood glucose control, high blood pressure, and high blood lipid levels.

The three distinct stages of diabetic retinopathy—nonproliferative, severe nonproliferative, and proliferative—are each defined by characteristic vision changes your doctor can detect with an ophthalmoscope. This instrument, which consists of a mirror that reflects light into the eye and a central hole through which the eye is examined, enables the doctor to view the interior structures of the eye, especially the retina.

Through frequent eye examinations, retinopathy can be detected and treated at its earliest stages, when the chances of safeguarding vision are improved. Identifying the specific stage of diabetic retinopathy is extremely important because the stage determines the treatment approach and how often follow-up visits should be scheduled.

Nonproliferative Retinopathy

In nonproliferative retinopathy, the blood vessels in the retina weaken and develop small bulges, called microaneurysms. Blood and hard exudates, composed of protein and fat in the retina, result from leaks from the damaged blood vessels and cause swelling of the retina.

Microaneurysms are the earliest changes that can be detected in a person with diabetic retinopathy. Through the ophthalmoscope, microaneurysms are seen as scattered red spots in the retina. Exudates appear as white or yellow areas, sometimes arranged in a ring around leaking capillaries (the minute blood vessels that link arteries to veins).

Nonproliferative retinopathy itself usually poses no danger to vision but rather serves as a warning sign that serious damage may later occur. Vision is impaired only when the swelling, bleeding, or exudates occur in the macula—a highly sensitive area at the center of the retina that is critical for fine vision. Swelling of the macula, called macular edema, can cause blurred vision and lead to visual loss.

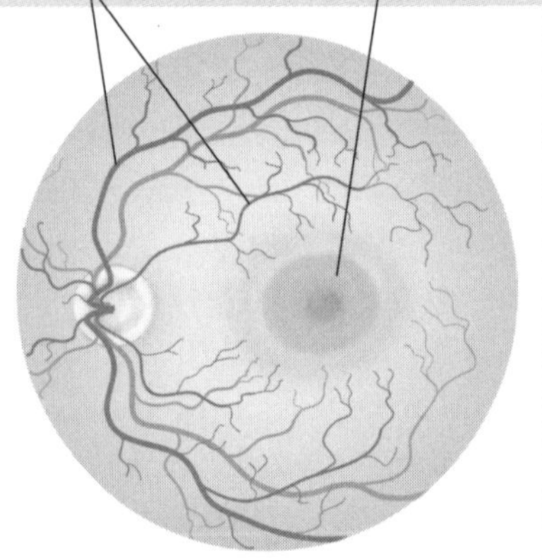

Normal eye

Regular eye examinations are important to detect any worsening of the retinopathy. Improved control of blood glucose (as well as blood pressure and lipid levels) may significantly reduce the risk of disease progression.

Severe Nonproliferative Retinopathy

Severe nonproliferative retinopathy (sometimes called preproliferative retinopathy) represents a more advanced stage of eye damage and is caused by decreased blood flow within the retina. In addition to the changes typically observed in nonproliferative retinopathy, this stage is marked by venous beading, cotton wool spots, and intraretinal microvascular abnormalities.

Venous beading initially consists of localized areas of dilation in small veins. The condition may progress to significant venous beading (a vein resembles a string of beads) and the formation of venous loops. Venous beading is considered an ominous sign because it strongly predicts the impending formation of new blood vessels, which are a hallmark of

Illustrations: Jacqueline Schaffer

blood glucose increases the risk of stroke because it changes the composition of blood lipoproteins, accelerates their oxidation, and thus makes them more likely to accumulate in the walls of arteries leading to the brain. In addition, high blood glucose levels may enhance the development of blood clots. But one of the most important risk factors for stroke is high blood pressure, which is

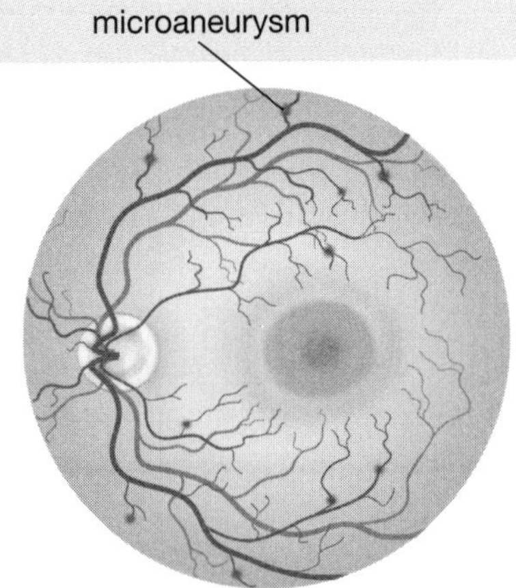

Nonproliferative diabetic retinopathy

proliferative retinopathy.

Cotton wool spots appear as soft white patches in the retina. The spots, which are usually larger than hard exudates and have less clearly defined margins, represent nerve damage resulting from blocked blood vessels.

Intraretinal microvascular abnormalities refer to irregularly shaped blood vessels that run between the normal vessels in the retina. These abnormal vessels appear as squiggly lines when viewed through the ophthalmoscope. Large numbers of intraretinal microvascular abnormalities predict the formation of new blood vessels.

Proliferative Retinopathy

Proliferative retinopathy is the most advanced stage of diabetic retinopathy. In this stage, abnormal new blood vessels proliferate on the surface of the retina and grow forward onto the back surface of the clear gel that fills the eyeball (the vitreous humor). Rupture of these fragile new blood vessels can cause bleeding into the vitreous humor. Such bleeding can block light from reaching the retina, causing blurred and distorted images and even temporary blindness.

Scar tissue may form on the retina if the bleeding is extensive or occurs repeatedly; it sometimes forms even in the absence of bleeding. By pulling the retina away from the back of the eye, such scarring can cause a retinal detachment. Left untreated, a retinal detachment can produce severe vision loss, or blindness.

A test called fluorescein angiography is often used to search for new blood vessels when their presence is suspected but they are not seen through the ophthalmoscope. In addition, the test can help determine whether vision loss is caused by macular ischemia (decreased blood flow to the macula) or macular edema. By locating leaking blood vessels, it can also serve as a guide for where to treat macular edema. In this test, fluorescein dye is injected into a vein in the arm, and a rapid series of photographs are taken of the retina as the dye passes through the blood vessels in the eye. The ophthalmologist then examines the photographs for signs of leakage of fluorescein dye from damaged blood vessels.

People with proliferative retinopathy are often unaware of the condition until a bleeding episode occurs. With regular eye exams, however, such new blood vessels can be detected early, and the use of laser photocoagulation therapy to seal the abnormal blood vessels can often prevent bleeding and vision deterioration.

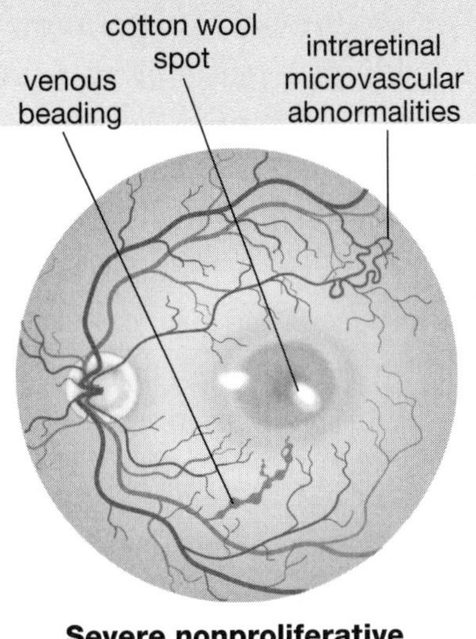

Severe nonproliferative diabetic retinopathy

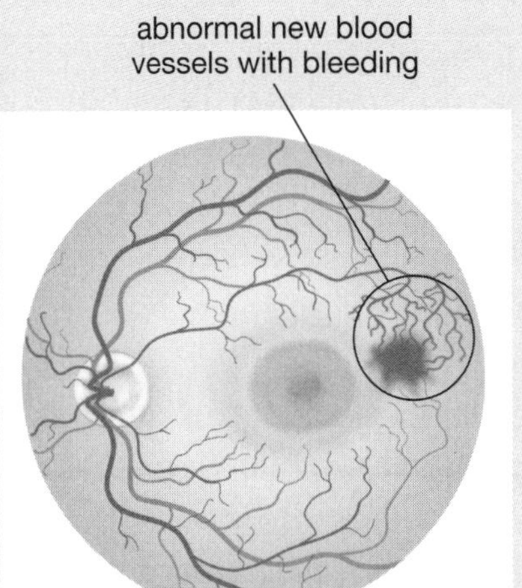

Proliferative diabetic retinopathy

approximately twice as common in patients with diabetes as in those without diabetes.

Peripheral vascular disease. Peripheral vascular disease is a narrowing of the arteries in the legs due to atherosclerosis. The characteristic symptom of peripheral vascular disease is intermittent claudication—pain in the thighs, calves, and sometimes the buttocks—that is brought on by exercise and goes away as soon as the exertion is stopped. In most people, pain occurs after a predictable amount of walking or running. Symptoms of peripheral vascular disease usually progress slowly over time, but eventually the pain can interfere with normal activities and may even occur at rest if blood vessels are severely narrowed. The poor blood supply associated with peripheral vascular disease can result in slow healing of foot blisters and other skin injuries, and may lead to chronic ulcer formation on the feet and legs.

Diabetes and cigarette smoking each double or triple the risk of peripheral vascular disease; since the effects are additive, a person with diabetes who smokes has an even greater risk. Preventive measures are directed toward correcting the same risk factors described for CHD. Severe symptoms of peripheral vascular disease can be treated with surgery to bypass the blocked vessels or with angioplasty, which compresses plaques using a small balloon inserted into the narrowed artery.

Diabetic Foot Problems

Normally, slight skin damage during the course of everyday activities creates minor pain in the feet that encourages an alteration in position or a change in gait. People with diabetes, however, may have diminished feeling in their legs and feet due to neuropathy. With the loss of pain sensation, these protective adjustments do not occur; trauma promotes skin breakdown and ulcer formation that may go unnoticed. Healing may be slowed or prevented because of a poor blood supply owing to atherosclerosis. If left untreated, foot damage may result in ulceration, infection, and even death of tissue (gangrene). Foot problems can often be avoided by performing a daily self-exam of the feet (see pages 51–52) and having a doctor examine the feet regularly.

TREATMENT OF DIABETES

The goals in the treatment of diabetes are to prevent its acute manifestations (high blood glucose and its symptoms of excessive thirst, frequent urination, and weight loss; hypoglycemia; diabetic ketoacidosis; and hyperosmolar coma) and its long-term complications (such as retinopathy, nephropathy, neuropathy, and macrovascular disease). Eating a healthful diet and exercising regularly are the first steps in treating diabetes, but some form of pharmacological treatment is often needed as well.

NEW RESEARCH

Statin Drug Shows Promise In Reducing Diabetes Risk

A statin drug used to reduce the risk of heart attack and stroke may also decrease the risk of type 2 diabetes, according to a new study.

Researchers from the United Kingdom analyzed data from 5,974 men (age 45 to 64) who participated in a study of the effectiveness of pravastatin (Pravachol), a lipid-lowering statin drug, for the prevention of coronary heart disease. About half of the participants received 40 mg of pravastatin a day; the other half received a placebo.

By the end of the six-year study, 139 men had developed type 2 diabetes. Participants who received pravastatin, however, had a 30% reduced risk of type 2 diabetes, compared with those who did not take the drug.

How pravastatin decreased the risk of diabetes in this study is not known. It is possible that the effect of pravastatin on the immune system—rather than its ability to lower lipid levels—may have played a role. By reducing inflammation, pravastatin may prevent or delay the onset of insulin resistance.

More research is needed to confirm these results and to determine whether they extend to other statin drugs. Pravastatin is not the only drug that has shown promise in the prevention of diabetes. In a recent study, the ACE inhibitor ramipril (Altace) decreased the risk of diabetes by about a third (see the sidebar on the opposite page).

CIRCULATION
Volume 103, page 357
January 23, 2001

The Diabetes Health Care Team

Many aspects of the proper management of diabetes necessarily depend on the actions of the patient. Because even basic health care is rendered more complicated by diabetes, it is best if people with the disorder work with a team of professionals who can provide the specialized medical knowledge necessary. Those members of the health care team with the initials C.D.E. after their names (for certified diabetes educator) have passed a special certification exam on patient education. The ADA can provide the names of certified diabetes educators in various localities. (See page 60 to contact the ADA.)

Some key members of a diabetes team include diabetes nurse educators, registered nurses who specialize in providing instruction and advice on issues related to the day-to-day management of diabetes; diabetes specialists, medical doctors such as diabetologists and endocrinologists; primary care physicians; nutritionists; registered dietitians; exercise physiologists to help people with diabetes create an individualized exercise program; mental health professionals; ophthalmologists; and podiatrists.

Control of Cardiovascular Disease Risk Factors

The high incidence of narrowing of the arteries (atherosclerosis) in diabetes demands strict attention to treatable risk factors: cigarette smoking; high blood pressure; high levels of LDL cholesterol, total cholesterol, and triglycerides; and low levels of HDL cholesterol. Several risk factors—including obesity, high blood pressure, high triglycerides, and low HDL cholesterol—are more common in people with diabetes than in the general population.

People with diabetes should strive for LDL cholesterol levels below 100 mg/dL, and HDL levels of 40 mg/dL or higher. Diet and, if necessary, drug therapy may be indicated in some cases to reach these levels.

High triglycerides (greater than 200 mg/dL) are best managed by weight loss and good control of diabetes, but drug treatment may be needed if patients fail to lose weight or if their triglycerides remain high despite weight loss and control of blood glucose.

Lifestyle changes are also effective in lowering the risk of cardiovascular complications. A recent study combined the results of several intervention trials that measured all causes of death in people with and without diabetes. Using statistical calculations, the analysis found that a 45-year-old man with diabetes would gain an average of one year of life expectancy with prophylactic aspirin

NEW RESEARCH

Antihypertensive Drug Reduces Diabetes Risk

The angiotensin converting enzyme (ACE) inhibitor ramipril (Altace) may help prevent diabetes in people at high risk for the disease, according to a recent study.

The study involved 5,720 individuals over age 55 who were taking part in the Heart Outcomes Prevention Evaluation (HOPE) trial. Participants had evidence of cardiovascular disease but were free of diabetes at the start of the trial.

Patients were randomly assigned to receive either ramipril (up to 10 mg/day) or a placebo. After an average follow-up period of 4.5 years, 102 people (3.6%) in the ramipril group developed diabetes compared with 155 (5.4%) in the placebo group—a greater than 30% reduction in risk with ramipril.

The investigators theorize that ACE inhibitors may protect against diabetes by slowing or reversing the decline in function of the pancreatic beta cells that produce insulin. The drugs may also reduce insulin resistance in muscle, liver, and fat cells.

Because of the "enormous clinical and public health potential" of the finding that ramipril appears to lower the risk of diabetes, these results require confirmation. Now underway is another trial evaluating ramipril and the antidiabetes drug rosiglitazone (Avandia) for diabetes prevention in people with impaired glucose tolerance.

JOURNAL OF THE AMERICAN MEDICAL ASSOCIATION
Volume 286, page 1882
October 17, 2001

treatment (to help prevent CHD) or with lower blood pressure, and gain over three years by quitting smoking. Several studies have shown that treatment with cholesterol-lowering drugs significantly reduces the risk of coronary events in people with diabetes who have a history of CHD. In the UKPDS (see below), modest reductions in blood pressure produced a striking decrease in cardiovascular events, such as heart attacks and strokes.

Tight Glucose Control

Control of blood glucose levels clearly prevents the symptoms of high blood glucose. Although doctors had long suspected that meticulous blood glucose control would slow or prevent the development of microvascular complications (retinopathy and nephropathy) and neuropathy, firm proof for this belief only became available in 1993, with the results from the DCCT, a 10-year study involving 1,441 men and women with type 1 diabetes. The participants followed one of two treatment regimens:

- Intensive treatment, which included monitoring of blood glucose levels three or four times a day, taking three or four insulin injections a day (or using an insulin pump), adjusting the insulin doses according to blood glucose levels, and following dietary and exercise recommendations daily; or
- Standard treatment, which involved daily glucose monitoring, one or two insulin injections a day, and following standard diet and exercise recommendations.

During the study, those in the intensive-treatment group had significantly lower fasting blood glucose and hemoglobin A1c levels than those in the standard-treatment group. Moreover, the intensive-treatment group reduced their risks of diabetic complications: retinopathy by 76%; neuropathy by 60%; and nephropathy by 35% to 56%. While this study included only individuals with type 1 diabetes, the recent findings of the UKPDS confirmed that improved glucose control provides similar protection against long-term microvascular complications in patients with type 2 diabetes. In the UKPDS, researchers followed 3,867 people with type 2 diabetes for 10 years. Half of the participants were randomly assigned to a conventional program starting with diet and exercise only; the rest were also treated with sulfonylurea drugs, metformin, and/or insulin. Compared to diet and exercise alone, drug therapy achieved better glucose control, resulting in a 25% reduction in retinopathy and kidney failure. A disappointing finding from the UKPDS was that improved blood glucose control with sulfonylurea or insulin

Is Tight Glucose Control Right for You?

The minimum goal of blood glucose control for all people with diabetes is to avoid the acute symptoms of high blood glucose—that is, excessive thirst, frequent urination, unintended weight loss, fatigue, ketoacidosis, and hyperosmolar nonketotic states (see pages 6–8). To achieve this goal, fasting blood glucose levels should generally be 200 mg/dL or lower. However, to reduce the risk of developing long-term complications from diabetes—neuropathy, retinopathy, and nephropathy—it is often recommended that patients maintain tight glucose control with a hemoglobin A1c level under 7%. Yet, for some elderly people, the risks of tight glucose control may outweigh the benefits. Consequently, the extent of blood glucose control should be individualized.

The main risk of glucose control that is too tight is hypoglycemia, which can lead to sweating, palpitations, fainting, double vision, confusion, and even coma. Some of these effects are of particular concern to older people who are at high risk for falls and subsequent disability. Nighttime hypoglycemia is also a serious concern for people who live alone and have no one to help them in the event of a hypoglycemic episode.

Life expectancy and general health status also should be taken into account when considering tight glucose control, which is meant to prevent complications that usually take 10 to 20 years to develop. Very old or very ill patients who have a limited life expectancy may not require strict control. Tight glucose control is more relevant to patients who are expected to live long enough to put themselves at risk for developing complications.

People with hypoglycemia unawareness—that is, an inability to recognize or feel the symptoms of a hypoglycemic reaction—should also have their blood glucose control targets relaxed. Studies have shown that awareness of hypoglycemia can be regained by preventing episodes of significant hypoglycemia for several months.

Tight glucose control may be dangerous for people who cannot or will not actively participate in the management of their condition. It may not be recommended for older people with a history of stroke or transient ischemic attacks, individuals with advanced diabetes complications, or people who take numerous medications for other illnesses that could interact with drugs used for glucose control.

Tight glucose control may not be practical for some older people who may have difficulty giving themselves insulin injections because of arthritis, poor vision, or cognitive impairment. Lastly, for people who have had diabetes for 20 to 25 years after puberty with minimal or no complications, a tightening of glucose control may not be needed because complications are unlikely to develop after this time.

only marginally reduced the incidence of cardiovascular events.

The accumulated evidence has led the ADA to conclude that all people with diabetes may benefit from better control of blood glucose levels. However, the ADA points out that aggressive blood glucose control might not be the right course of action for everyone. The participants in the intensive-treatment group of the DCCT had a three-times higher incidence of hypoglycemia, which can be more dangerous in people who are older or have cardiovascular disease. (For more information on the benefits and risks of

NEW FINDING

Markers of Inflammation May Help Identify People at Risk for Diabetes

Women with the highest levels of C-reactive protein (CRP) or interleukin-6 (IL-6) are at increased risk for type 2 diabetes, according to the findings of a recent report from the Women's Health Study.

The 27,628 women in the study were free of diabetes, cardiovascular disease, and cancer at the start of the study. Researchers compared 188 women who developed type 2 diabetes over a four-year period with a control group of 362 women who did not develop diabetes during that time.

The women with the highest levels of CRP at the beginning of the study were 15.7 times more likely to develop diabetes than those with the lowest levels. Similarly, women with the highest IL-6 levels were 7.5 times more likely to develop diabetes than those with the lowest levels.

Because elevated levels of CRP and IL-6 signal the presence of inflammation in the body, these findings support a possible role for inflammation in the development of diabetes. The authors suggest that measurements of inflammatory markers such as CRP might aid in the early detection of individuals at increased risk for the disease.

JOURNAL OF THE AMERICAN MEDICAL ASSOCIATION
Volume 286, page 327
July 18, 2001

tight glucose control, see the feature on page 23.)

Nevertheless, people with diabetes—whether they have type 1 or type 2—should strive for the best blood glucose control that is safely possible. No explicit guidelines have been set for tight control, and targets will vary from person to person. The intensive-care group in the DCCT achieved an average blood glucose level of around 155 mg/dL. While tight control always involves blood glucose monitoring, it may not require insulin injections in individuals with type 2 diabetes: A carefully constructed program of diet, exercise, and oral drugs, if needed, may suffice.

Self-Monitoring of Blood Glucose Control

Currently, the best method to assess diabetic control is self-testing of blood glucose. (Testing for the presence of glucose in the urine is far less useful.) Results from the DCCT and other recent studies indicate that people with diabetes must be more aggressive in their daily monitoring of blood glucose levels. This means not only making more frequent measurements, but also adjusting diet, exercise, and doses of insulin or oral diabetes drugs according to the results.

Along with regularly measuring blood glucose levels, people with diabetes should keep a log of their readings. (A log book is often included with the purchase of a blood glucose meter.) This record allows more accurate tracking of progress and can help point out the source of difficulties in controlling diabetes. Thus, if high or low blood glucose levels follow a trend—occurring several days in a row at the same time each day—reviewing the log with a doctor can lead to suggestions on changing medication, or adjusting the timing or dose of insulin. In some cases, unexpected fluctuations in blood glucose readings can be traced to simple changes in routine, for example, eating unusually large or small meals, variations in exercise, or even psychological stress.

An even better way for health care professionals to evaluate results is to download the glucose readings from the meter into a computer. Patterns often become clear when the downloaded information is displayed on a printout.

Blood glucose testing. The development of simple and accurate tests to measure blood glucose, which allow people with diabetes to make rapid changes in their diet and medication, has made home glucose monitoring the backbone of diabetic management. Most blood tests require only a single drop of blood, which can be withdrawn by a special lancet or by the meter itself in some cases. (A wide variety of devices can make drawing blood as painless and simple as possible; some are spring-loaded and adjustable to give as shallow a stick as possible while still drawing blood.)

The blood is then placed on a reagent strip impregnated with an enzyme called glucose oxidase. The blood glucose level is determined by inserting the strip into a meter, which provides a digital readout. (The older method of visually comparing the color of the strip to a chart is far less accurate.) The meters take from 15 to 45 seconds to give a result. Recommendations for the frequency and timing of glucose monitoring vary from once a day or less in patients with very stable, well controlled type 2 diabetes to multiple times daily in type 1 patients.

There are many different types of glucose monitors with a large number of features. A doctor or diabetes educator can provide information on the type of monitor best suited to individual needs. Factors to be considered are whether the numbers on the readout can be read easily, how difficult the meter is to use, and whether it has advanced memory features that could simplify record keeping. Monitors that can download meter results and print out summaries are particularly useful. The test strips required by the meter should also be considered. Since the strips are perishable, they come packaged either in a vial or individually wrapped in foil, which might be difficult to handle for people with arthritis.

Prices for the meter (ranging from $30 to about $130) can be greatly reduced through rebates and special offers from manufacturers; most companies offer discounts because only their brand of test strips can be used in their meter, and the test strips are expensive. In fact, over time the cost of the strips is far greater than the cost of the meter itself. Some insurance companies do reimburse for certain meters and strips, and this should be investigated before making a purchase.

In the past few years, the U.S. Food and Drug Administration (FDA) has approved several new methods for testing blood glucose. The FreeStyle blood glucose monitoring system (TheraSense, Inc.), the One Touch FastTake system (LifeScan, Inc.), and the Precision Xtra (MediSense) require blood samples, while the GlucoWatch Biographer (Cygnus, Inc.) is a noninvasive monitor that analyzes glucose by collecting fluid through the skin without piercing it.

FreeStyle. The advantage of the FreeStyle blood glucose monitoring system is that blood can be drawn from the forearm, which is less sensitive than the fingers. The system requires only 0.3 microliters of blood, a drop the size of a pinhead.

To use FreeStyle, the patient inserts a test strip into the hand-

NEW RESEARCH

Accurate Readings Obtained With New Glucose Monitoring Device

In a study of a new blood glucose monitor that draws blood from the arm rather than a finger, researchers found that the device provided accurate blood glucose readings.

To use the device, called the Sof-Tac Diabetes Management System, the patient places it on the forearm or upper arm and presses a button. The device then creates a vacuum seal against the skin, releases a lancet, and draws blood into a test strip. Blood glucose results are provided in 40 seconds from the time the device is placed on the arm.

In a study conducted by the manufacturers of the device, 378 people (both with and without diabetes), age 18 to 84, were asked to follow the device's instructions and test their blood glucose. Health care professionals then used the device to test the participants' blood glucose. Afterward, finger-stick testing was performed by both the participants and health care professionals.

There were no significant differences between blood glucose readings taken from the arm with the new device and those from the finger-stick method, or between readings performed by health care professionals and participants. Most participants reported that the device was less painful than the finger-stick method.

DIABETES CARE
Volume 24, page 1217
July 2001

held glucose monitor, pricks the forearm lightly with a lancet, and touches the edge of the strip to the blood sample. The monitor produces a blood glucose reading in an average of 15 seconds. The meter itself costs $75; the test strips are about $40 for a package of 50. Lancets cost about $10 for a package of 100.

One Touch FastTake. The One Touch FastTake system is similar to FreeStyle in that patients can draw blood from the forearm and receive results in about 15 seconds. Its memory records up to 150 tests, including the date, time, and a 14-day average reading. The meter goes for approximately $60, and the test strips cost around $40 for a package of 50. A package of 100 lancets costs around $9.

Precision Xtra. The Precision Xtra meter has a unique feature: It allows patients to monitor not only glucose, but ketone levels as well. The only other way to monitor ketone levels at home is through urine tests. The ability to test blood ketone levels quickly can help to prevent diabetic ketoacidosis, which can occur when blood glucose levels rise above 300 mg/dL.

Precision Xtra is similar in size to other personal blood glucose meters. It requires a blood sample of 5 microliters taken from the finger and produces a glucose reading in about 20 seconds. Ketone readings take around 30 seconds. The meter itself costs about $90, and test strips cost $68 for a package of 100. The lancing device is part of the meter itself.

GlucoWatch Biographer. The GlucoWatch Biographer, a device worn on the wrist, can determine glucose levels through intact skin. The back of the watch sends a low electrical current through the skin, which draws glucose-containing fluid from adjacent cells, not from the blood. After a three-hour warm-up period and an initial calibration with a traditional fingerstick, GlucoWatch can provide a glucose reading every 20 minutes for 12 hours. GlucoWatch can supplement standard glucose measurements, but it does not replace them; users still need to perform a finger-stick test before injecting insulin.

The device costs about $300 and is designed to last for two to three years. The sensors for the back of the watch last for 12 hours after calibration and cost $4 or more.

Urine glucose testing. When glucose builds up to a certain level in the blood, the excess begins to "spill over" into the urine. This typically occurs at blood glucose levels exceeding 180 mg/dL, or 200 mg/dL in older adults. Testing urine for the presence of glucose provides a rough idea of diabetic control; however, it is far less useful than blood glucose monitoring. Test strips are passed

The Dangers of High-Protein, Low-Carbohydrate Diets for People With Diabetes

Maintaining a healthy body weight is important for both the prevention and treatment of diabetes. Excess body weight increases the risk of developing diabetes; and for overweight people with the disease, losing weight can improve blood glucose control and reduce the risk of long-term complications.

Losing weight is difficult, however, and many people resort to fad diets. Among the most popular ones today are high-protein, low-carbohydrate diets that promise rapid weight loss by following a food plan that is high in protein but limits foods rich in carbohydrates, such as fruits, vegetables, and grains. Some examples are *Dr. Atkins' New Diet Revolution* by Robert C. Atkins, M.D., *Protein Power* by Michael R. Eades, M.D. and Mary Dan Eades, M.D., *Sugar Busters!* by H. Leighton Steward, M.S. and coauthors, and *The Zone* by Barry Sears, Ph.D. According to the authors of these diets, high levels of insulin cause obesity by promoting the storage of calories as body fat. They claim that when a person reduces the amount of carbohydrate in the diet, the body produces less insulin and weight loss occurs.

People do lose weight on high-protein, low-carbohydrate diets, though the weight loss is due to water loss and reduced calories, not to lower insulin levels as the authors claim. Even so, nutrition experts do not recommend these diets. First, the weight loss is difficult to maintain over the long term. Second, there is some evidence that these diets may increase the risk of coronary heart disease (CHD) and kidney damage—conditions for which people with diabetes are already at high risk.

Weight Loss Is Difficult To Maintain

High-protein, low-carbohydrate diets may produce greater weight loss than other diets. But this weight loss is mostly water—rather than fat—and weight is quickly regained when you go off the diet. Why? A decreased intake of carbohydrates depletes carbohydrate stores in your body, and the water associated with these stores is released from the body. When you start eating carbohydrates again, the water returns. In addition, because high-protein, low-carbohydrate diets restrict food choices, people cannot follow these diets for long periods of time, and the lost weight is ultimately regained.

Increased Risk of Coronary Heart Disease

Diets high in protein tend to be high in fat, particularly saturated fat. For example, the Atkins diet and *Protein Power* provide about 20% to 25% of calories from saturated fat. In comparison, the American Diabetes Association recommends that less than 10% of calories come from this type of fat.

Diets high in saturated fat can raise blood cholesterol levels, which in turn increase the risk of CHD. In a study of the Atkins diet, published in the *Journal of the American Dietetic Association* in September 1980, people who followed the diet for eight weeks experienced an increase in blood cholesterol levels, even though they had lost weight. (Weight loss is known to decrease cholesterol levels.) In a more recent study in the October 2000 issue of the *Journal of the American College of Nutrition,* researchers calculated that long-term use of the Atkins diet would result in a 25% increase in blood cholesterol levels, which translates to an increased risk of CHD of more than 50%.

High-protein, low-carbohydrate diets can also increase your risk of CHD because they tend to be low in fiber, owing to the restrictions on fruits, vegetables, and grains. While the American Diabetes Association recommends 20 to 35 g of fiber per day, the Atkins diet and *Protein Power* supply only 5 to 10 g. Research shows that foods high in soluble fiber, such as oat bran, legumes, and apples, can decrease cholesterol levels and protect against CHD.

Increased Risk of Kidney Dysfunction

The American Diabetes Association recommends that people with diabetes consume no more than 20% of calories from protein. High-protein, low-carbohydrate diets exceed these recommendations: Protein makes up 35% of the calories in the Atkins diet and *Protein Power,* and 28% of the calories in *Sugar Busters* and *The Zone.* Such high levels of protein may increase the risk of kidney damage in people with diabetes and exacerbate existing kidney disease.

Another way that high-protein, low-carbohydrate diets may cause kidney problems is through a process called ketosis. Ketosis, which occurs when you do not eat enough carbohydrates, results in the production of acidic substances known as ketones that may build up in the bloodstream in people with type 1 diabetes. This can lead to a diabetic emergency known as diabetic ketoacidosis.

The Best Weight Loss Plan

The best way to lose weight—and to keep it off—is not to look for a "quick fix," but to make lifestyle changes that involve reducing the total amount of calories you eat while increasing your level of physical activity. Remember, it is excess calories, not excess carbohydrates, that make you fat.

So eat a variety of foods to ensure that you get all the essential nutrients that your body needs. By choosing foods that are higher in carbohydrates and fiber and lower in fat, you can also improve blood glucose control and decrease your risk of CHD and kidney damage.

through the urine stream or have drops of urine placed on them. The presence of glucose in the urine causes a color change in the tablet or strip. The color is then compared to a chart to determine roughly how much glucose is present.

Because urine tests are positive for glucose only when the blood glucose level is over 180 to 200 mg/dL, these tests cannot detect more moderate glucose elevations or hypoglycemia. In addition, there is a lag from the time when the blood glucose level is excessive until the time when it is found in the urine. Thus, anyone attempting to keep their blood glucose levels within a set range would be acting on late and incomplete information. Also, urine glucose measurements can be affected by intake of vitamin C, aspirin, and fluids, as well as by incomplete emptying of the bladder prior to taking the test. For these reasons, urine glucose testing is rarely recommended.

Ketone testing. Ketone bodies in the urine can be measured easily by placing a test strip or tablet in urine and examining it for a color change. Typically, only people with type 1 diabetes need to perform this test. A person should check for ketones if blood glucose levels are over 250 mg/dL and symptoms such as fruity breath, nausea, vomiting, or difficulties in concentration suggest ketoacidosis. If the test is strongly positive, a doctor should be called immediately.

Dietary Measures

The right diet may not only keep glucose levels in check but also help to control a number of other factors, such as elevated blood lipids, obesity, and high blood pressure, that affect the risk of developing diabetic complications.

Most experts recommend that people with diabetes eat a high-carbohydrate/low-fat diet. According to this school of thought, 50% to 60% of calories should come from carbohydrates and 30% or fewer from fat. The primary goal of this diet is to keep blood lipid levels low—so as to reduce the risk of macrovascular disease—without adversely affecting blood glucose levels. Most people do best when they consume a relatively stable amount of carbohydrates at each meal, rather than trying to eliminate carbohydrates, which increases the amount of fat in the diet.

For people with diabetes, as for everyone, it is important to control the intake of total calories, saturated fat, and cholesterol. Weight loss is extremely important for those who are overweight. It not only improves control of blood glucose and blood pressure, but may also lower total cholesterol, raise HDL cholesterol, and reduce elevated triglyceride levels.

The most effective way to lose weight is to combine a lower caloric intake with exercise. This combination not only produces faster and more permanent weight loss, but also prevents excessive loss of muscle mass (which burns more calories even at rest) and strengthens the cardiovascular system. Approximately 1 lb of body weight is lost for every 3,500 calories of reduced caloric intake or increased energy expended in physical activity. Highly regimented popular diets work temporarily for many people but are usually extremely difficult to sustain. Ultimately, such rigid diets need to be transformed into more balanced, healthy, and sustainable dietary habits.

Saturated fat raises blood cholesterol levels and should make up no more than 10% of total calories. To lower LDL cholesterol to the goal of less than 100 mg/dL, people with diabetes may need to restrict their intake of saturated fat to 7% of total calories. Some studies have found that saturated fat may also elevate blood insulin levels, which could contribute to CHD. In one study of 652 men without diabetes, reducing saturated fat intake from 14% to 8% of calories lowered fasting insulin levels by 18% and post-meal insulin levels by 25%.

Although dietary cholesterol has a smaller impact on blood lipid levels than saturated fat, people with diabetes should still limit their intake to no more than 200 mg each day.

Rather than calculating the percent of calories from saturated fat and counting milligrams of cholesterol, it may be easier simply to cut back on foods high in these substances. Foods high in saturated fat include red meats, dark meat poultry, poultry skin, whole-milk dairy products, butter, and products made with hydrogenated oils or coconut, palm, or palm kernel oils. Cholesterol is found only in animal products, and is particularly plentiful in egg yolks, organ meats, shrimp, crab, and lobster.

Another way to reduce saturated fat in the diet is to replace it with monounsaturated fat. Monounsaturated fat—which is plentiful in olive oil, canola oil, avocados, and some nuts—lowers total blood cholesterol levels without reducing HDL cholesterol levels. (Polyunsaturated fat lowers total cholesterol levels, but may also reduce HDL cholesterol levels.) Furthermore, the substitution of monounsaturated fat for polyunsaturated fat in the diet decreases the likelihood of LDL oxidation, which is now thought to initiate the accumulation of LDL cholesterol in the walls of arteries—a precursor to atherosclerosis.

NEW RESEARCH

Diet and Exercise Help Prevent Diabetes in People at High Risk

Lifestyle changes can help people at high risk for type 2 diabetes lower their chances of developing the disease, according to a recent clinical trial.

The Diabetes Prevention Program was conducted at 27 medical centers nationwide, including Johns Hopkins, and involved 3,234 participants. All were overweight and had impaired glucose tolerance, which means their blood glucose levels were higher than normal but not at diabetic levels.

Participants were randomly assigned to treatment with metformin (Glucophage), a placebo, or lifestyle changes that included a low-fat diet and 150 minutes of exercise per week. The participants were followed for an average of three years.

The group assigned to lifestyle changes lost an average of 15 lbs and lowered their risk of diabetes by 58%. Lifestyle changes were most effective in people over age 60, who reduced their risk of developing diabetes by 71%.

In the metformin group, the risk of diabetes was lowered by 31%. However, metformin, which is normally used to treat rather than prevent diabetes, had little effect in participants who were older or less overweight. Researchers did not study the potential benefits of combining metformin with diet and exercise.

U.S. DEPARTMENT OF HEALTH AND HUMAN SERVICES ANNOUNCEMENT
August 6, 2001

Other dietary considerations in diabetes include the following.

Dietary fiber. By slowing the absorption of sugars from the intestine, dietary fiber diminishes the rise in blood glucose that follows the ingestion of carbohydrates. Some studies have shown that an increase in soluble fiber—found in oats, oat bran, legumes, barley, citrus fruits, and apples—can help lower blood glucose and cholesterol levels. Insoluble fiber—found in whole wheat, wheat bran, vegetables, and fruit—can help prevent constipation. Both types of fiber are needed for a healthy diet. Ideally, 25 to 40 g of dietary fiber should be consumed each day.

Sugar. In its latest recommendations, the ADA appeared to relax its previous restrictions on sugar (sucrose) intake for people with diabetes. This change was made because, when eaten in exactly the same amounts, sweets and complex carbohydrates (starches) affect blood glucose levels similarly. The problem is that a small portion of sweets equals the carbohydrate content of a much larger serving of complex carbohydrates. Therefore, it is preferable for people with diabetes to avoid sugar-containing foods because it is easy to ingest far too many calories from carbohydrates when eating sweets. (For more information on sugar, see the feature on the opposite page.)

Antioxidants. Antioxidants are chemical compounds that help prevent cell damage by inactivating molecules called free radicals that are formed during the normal course of metabolism. Though animal and population studies suggest that the antioxidant vitamin E may diminish the risk of macrovascular disease by protecting LDL from oxidation, in two large trials, vitamin supplements did not prevent cardiovascular events in people with known coronary heart disease or diabetes with other risk factors.

Sodium. Patients with high blood pressure should restrict their sodium intake to less than 2,500 mg per day by using less salt at the table and in cooking, and by avoiding foods that are high in sodium (for example, processed meats such as sausages, cured ham, and hot dogs; canned or dried soups; ketchup; and most cheeses).

Protein. About 10% to 20% of calories should come from protein. Most experts now agree that reducing dietary protein slows further kidney damage in those with diabetic nephropathy. Diets billed as "high protein" should be viewed with caution. (For more information on the dangers of high-protein diets, see the feature on page 27.)

Alcohol. People with well controlled diabetes can drink alcoholic beverages in moderation and with food. The ADA recommends that men drink no more than two alcoholic drinks per day,

ESSAY

Can People With Diabetes Include Sugar In Their Diet?

by Christopher D. Saudek, M.D.

One of the most common questions in considering a nutritional plan for diabetes is, "Can I eat sugar?" Surprisingly, after all these years, the answer remains confusing and even controversial. Why is this the case? Because the academic, scientific answer may not match the practical, behavioral answer. So what are the facts, and what is a person to do?

The fact is that when a person with type 1 or type 2 diabetes ingests concentrated sweets (such as candy, pies, cakes, and doughnuts), their blood glucose may rise a bit more quickly, but not necessarily any more, than if the person ate *an equal number of grams* of a complex carbohydrate such as potatoes or rice. Based on these sorts of observations, which were done on patients in a hospital research ward, both the American Diabetes Association and the Canadian Diabetes Association now state in their recommendations that people with diabetes may consume some of their total calories from sugar or sweets.

So what's the problem with eating sweets? Simply, it is that most people just *add* sweets, they don't *substitute* them for exactly the same amount of complex carbohydrate. For example, if you have a doughnut at the office (approximately 45 g of carbohydrate), do you eliminate three slices of bread from lunch? If you have a 3½" piece of apple pie (estimated at 75 g of carbohydrate), do you eliminate two medium baked potatoes from dinner? Another problem: do you really know how many carbohydrates were in that doughnut or piece of pie?

For these reasons, I caution against sweets for people with diabetes. At best, they are empty calories, devoid of nutritional value; at worst, they can wreak havoc on your blood glucose control.

It's not all doom and denial, though. If people with diabetes decide to incorporate a certain amount of sugar or sweets into their diet, they should do so carefully and with their eyes wide open. The best way to make it easy and predictable is to be consistent: Have a small dessert such as a scoop of ice cream or a cookie after your regular supper, take the right amount of insulin or oral medication, and then check your blood glucose several hours later. If your blood glucose is okay, you will know that you can tolerate a small dessert after supper.

But remember it is easy to ingest far too many calories when eating sweets. If you do eat sugar-containing foods, remember to eat fewer carbohydrates at your next meal and to get some exercise to burn off the extra calories.

In addition, many sugar-containing foods, like ice cream and cookies, are high in fat. If you choose to eat a sugar-containing food, seek out low-fat sweets, like graham crackers, fig bars, or low-fat frozen yogurt. Keep in mind, however, that many low-fat versions of products like ice cream often replace fat with sugar.

In the end, the most important thing is to work with an experienced dietitian to develop a meal plan that is satisfying and good for you as an individual.

and women no more than one. Alcohol should not be consumed on an empty stomach by people who take insulin or oral blood glucose-lowering drugs. People with additional medical problems, such as pancreatitis (inflammation of the pancreas) or elevated triglyceride levels, should abstain altogether.

The calories from alcohol should be exchanged for those that would normally be allotted for fat servings. Drinks that contain smaller amounts of sugar, such as light beers and dry wines, are preferable to mixed drinks that are high in sugar.

Heavy drinking should be avoided, and those who drink should be aware that alcohol can cause weight gain (because of its high caloric content), hypoglycemia, elevated triglycerides, and flushing or nausea in some people taking oral diabetes drugs, especially chlorpropamide (Diabinese).

Exercise

While it is probable that exercise helps to prevent diabetes, it is certain that regular exercise benefits those who already have the disorder. Exercise may be limited by arthritis, CHD, or peripheral vascular disease, and those with peripheral neuropathy may need to modify their type of workout to avoid foot trauma (for example, by replacing running with swimming).

Exercise burns calories and thus helps control weight, and can also lower blood glucose levels by enhancing insulin action. In addition, exercise may postpone or eliminate the long-term complications of the disease. For example, exercise can lower blood pressure and triglycerides while raising HDL cholesterol. Furthermore, a 2000 study of 1,263 men with type 2 diabetes (average age 50) found that the men who were least fit were twice as likely to die after 12 years as the men who were most fit.

Though physical activity can be increased by changing everyday habits, such as taking the stairs rather than an elevator, it is more effective to set aside time for exercise (even a simple program of brisk walks) on a regular basis. Those taking insulin must know, however, that the enhanced insulin action produced by vigorous exercise can cause hypoglycemia (sometimes not until 8 to 12 hours afterward).

Oral Agents to Lower Blood Glucose

Diet and exercise may suffice to control blood glucose levels in some patients with type 2 diabetes; but when the response to these measures is inadequate, oral agents are generally started.

The six classes of oral agents are the sulfonylureas, biguanides, alpha-glucosidase inhibitors, meglitinides, thiazolidinediones, and D-phenylalanine derivatives, the most recently-approved class. Each class acts on different parts of the body and through different mechanisms to lower blood glucose levels. (The feature on page 35 and the chart on pages 36–37 provide an overview of these drugs.)

Sulfonylureas. The sulfonylureas available in the United States are classified as first-generation or second-generation. Chlorpropamide (Diabinese) is a first-generation sulfonylurea. Second-generation drugs include glimepiride (Amaryl), glipizide (Glucotrol) and its widely used extended-release formulation (Glucotrol XL), and glyburide (DiaBeta, Glynase, Micronase). Doses of the second-generation drugs are much smaller than those for the first-generation agents. They all have similar chemical structures and modes of action (they all stimulate the pancreas to secrete insulin). Therefore, if a person loses responsiveness to one sulfonylurea (which often happens), a drug from another class may be added or substituted. Switching to another sulfonylurea is not likely to help.

About 85% of patients with type 2 diabetes who have not responded adequately to diet initially show a favorable response to sulfonylureas. Specifically, most patients with fasting glucose levels below 250 mg/dL show some response to these drugs; those with fasting glucose levels above 300 mg/dL rarely respond to them. In more than one quarter of patients with an initially good response, these drugs lose their effectiveness. When sulfonylureas do not lower blood glucose levels sufficiently, metformin or a thiazolidinedione can be added. Alternately, metformin alone may be tried as a replacement. A combination of glyburide and metformin called Glucovance is now available. If all types of oral agents fail, insulin is used.

Adverse side effects occur in roughly 3% of patients. The most common and serious side effect is hypoglycemia, which is more likely to occur in debilitated elderly patients, malnourished individuals, and those with abnormalities of pituitary, adrenal, liver, or kidney function. Alcohol ingestion, skipped meals, and exercise can also trigger hypoglycemia when taking a sulfonylurea. If hypoglycemia occurs, the dose of sulfonylurea is usually reduced. The sulfonylurea drug chlorpropamide can cause excessive water retention, thus lowering the blood sodium level. In addition, chlorpropamide may occasionally cause severe headaches and flushing after drinking alcohol.

Biguanides. Several years ago, the FDA approved another drug—metformin (Glucophage), which belongs to a class of oral agents called the biguanides. An extended-release form of the drug became available in 2000. Metformin works alone or in conjunction with sulfonylurea drugs to lower blood glucose. Some studies have shown that it can reduce blood glucose levels by about 20% on its own, and boost the glucose-lowering effects of a sulfonylurea by an additional 25%. It acts primarily by decreasing the liver's glucose production but also increases the uptake of glucose by muscles.

One of metformin's main attractions is that it provides another option for type 2 diabetes patients who do not achieve adequate glucose control with a sulfonylurea. In fact, metformin can be used either as the first-line oral agent (before a sulfonylurea), or as a second-line agent when the sulfonylureas no longer work adequately. Additional benefits include a significant reduction in cholesterol and triglycerides. Patients on metformin alone do not develop hypoglycemia or gain weight (they may even lose some), in contrast to those treated with sulfonylureas or insulin. In one study, metformin

NEW RESEARCH

Exercise and Risk of Cardiovascular Disease in People With Diabetes

Exercise is associated with a decreased risk of heart disease and stroke in the general population. Does the same hold true for people with type 2 diabetes? To find out, researchers studied 5,125 female nurses with type 2 diabetes over a period of 14 years.

The results showed that exercise was associated with a lower risk of heart disease and stroke in these diabetic nurses. Among women who walked for exercise, those who walked the farthest and the fastest had a 34% lower risk of heart disease and stroke than those who walked the least. For women who engaged in more vigorous physical activity, greater reductions in risk were observed in those who spent larger amounts of time exercising each week. For example, women who performed moderate or vigorous exercise at least four hours a week had about a 40% lower risk than those who exercised less than one hour per week.

This study provides further evidence for the benefits of exercise in people with type 2 diabetes. However, exercise must be undertaken with caution in these individuals because of the possibility of hypoglycemia and other complications. Consult your doctor before initiating an exercise program.

ANNALS OF INTERNAL MEDICINE
Volume 134, page 96
January 16, 2001

helped patients to lose an average of almost 6 lbs, most of which (88%) was body fat. The weight loss may be due to a small decrease in appetite experienced by patients taking the drug.

The most common side effect of metformin is diarrhea, which tends to resolve on its own even with continued use of the drug. Other side effects include mild nausea, bloating, and gas. These gastrointestinal side effects occur in 30% of patients. Metformin can also cause hypoglycemia when used in combination with a sulfonylurea or insulin. A buildup of lactic acid in the blood (lactic acidosis) is rare but is life-threatening should it occur. To avoid this dangerous complication, metformin should not be used in people with kidney or liver disease, heart failure, severe emphysema or other chronic lung diseases, or heavy alcohol intake.

Alpha-glucosidase inhibitors. Acarbose (Precose) and miglitol (Glyset), which inhibit alpha-glucosidase enzymes in the intestine, are taken just before meals. By delaying the digestion of complex carbohydrates and sucrose (table sugar), they blunt the peak levels of blood glucose and insulin after a meal. The most common side effects—gas, diarrhea, and abdominal discomfort—tend to lessen over time, but many patients are unable to tolerate these drugs because of excessive gas.

Acarbose and miglitol should not be used by people with inflammatory bowel disease or other serious intestinal disorders. The drugs can be taken in combination with sulfonylureas, metformin, or the thiazolidinediones. The drugs alone do not cause hypoglycemia. If hypoglycemia occurs when taking both a sulfonylurea and acarbose or miglitol, the condition must be treated by ingesting glucose (dextrose) or fruit juice (fruit juices contain sugars that do not need to be digested) rather than products containing cane sugar (sucrose), which cannot be digested and absorbed due to the effects of acarbose and miglitol.

Meglitinides. Repaglinide (Prandin) works by a different mechanism than sulfonylureas to induce pancreatic insulin secretion (in a way that is dependent on the amount of glucose in the blood). Repaglinide has a more rapid effect on insulin levels, and so may offer more flexibility than sulfonylureas. It can be taken from 30 minutes to immediately before each meal; the drug is not used when meals are not eaten.

Repaglinide can be taken in combination with metformin if either drug alone does not control blood glucose adequately. Hypoglycemia was the most common side effect found in studies of this drug. Dosages range from 0.5 to 4 mg with each meal. In one study,

Oral Medications for Type 2 Diabetes

While type 1 diabetes is caused by a lack of insulin production and has a relatively straightforward treatment (insulin injections), the management of type 2 diabetes is more complex. Type 2 diabetes results when the body's cells are not sensitive enough to the effects of insulin and cannot take in enough glucose from the blood, the pancreas produces insufficient insulin to compensate for this insulin insensitivity, the liver releases too much glucose, or a combination of these factors. Six classes of oral drugs are available to treat type 2 diabetes; each acts on different sites in the body and through different mechanisms to control blood glucose levels (see the illustration below). These drugs should be used in conjunction with diet and exercise and are only effective if the pancreas produces insulin (making them ineffective for people with type 1 diabetes). They may be prescribed individually, in combination, or (later in the disease) with insulin.

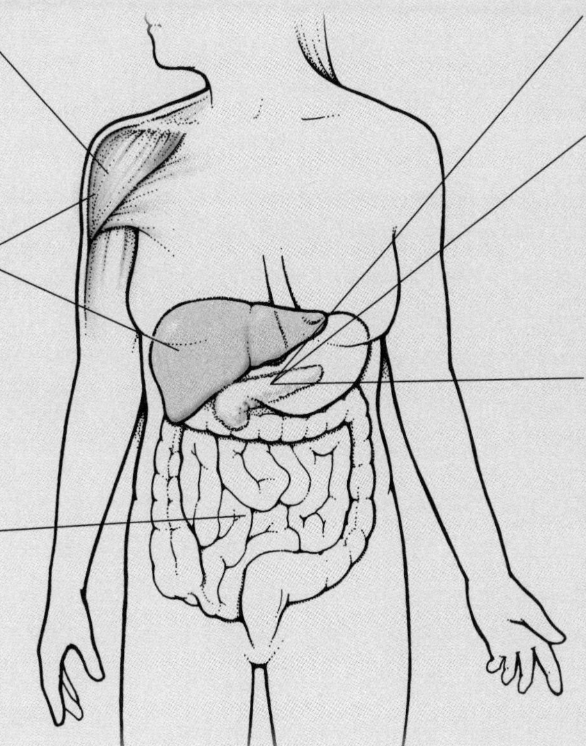

patients taking repaglinide demonstrated significantly better glucose control than those using a placebo. During the study, hemoglobin A1c levels dropped from 8.5% to 7.8% with repaglinide, compared with an increase from 8.1% to 9.3% with a placebo. The drug was generally well tolerated, although 36% of users reported mild to moderate hypoglycemic symptoms.

Thiazolidinediones heighten the sensitivity of muscle and fat cells to insulin, increasing the body's response to the insulin produced by the pancreas.
The biguanide metformin decreases glucose levels in the blood primarily by lowering glucose production in the liver. It also increases the uptake of glucose by muscle cells.
Alpha-glucosidase inhibitors block the activity of enzymes in the intestine that convert carbohydrates into simple sugars (such as glucose). This minimizes the increase in blood glucose that usually occurs after a meal.
Sulfonylureas act to stimulate the pancreas to produce more insulin.
Meglitinides, like sulfonylureas, stimulate the pancreas to release more insulin. Meglitinides are taken shortly before eating and lower the rise in blood glucose that normally follows a meal.
The D-phenylalanine derivative nateglinide, like sulfonylureas and meglitinides, stimulates the pancreas to release more insulin. Nateglinide is chemically different from these drugs and has a distinct mechanism of action, however. Nateglinide is taken shortly before eating and lowers the rise in blood glucose that normally follows a meal.

Thiazolidinediones. Rosiglitazone (Avandia) and pioglitazone (Actos) are the two drugs available from this relatively new (and expensive) class of oral glucose-lowering drugs. The thiazolidinediones work by decreasing resistance of muscle cells to insulin. Since obese people with diabetes are resistant to insulin, they may

Oral Blood Glucose-Lowering Agents 2002

Drug Type	Generic Name	Brand Name	Onset and Duration of Action
Sulfonylureas	chlorpropamide	Diabinese	Should be taken once a day with breakfast; peaks in 2 to 4 hours and lasts for 24 to 28 hours.
	glimepiride	Amaryl	Should be taken once a day with breakfast; peaks in 2 to 3 hours and lasts for 24 hours.
	glipizide	Glucotrol	Should be taken once or twice a day 30 minutes before a meal; peaks in 1 to 3 hours and lasts 12 to 24 hours.
	glipizide, extended-release	Glucotrol XL	Should be taken once a day with breakfast; peaks in 6 to 12 hours and lasts for 24 hours.
	glyburide	DiaBeta Glynase Micronase	Should be taken once or twice a day before a meal; peaks in 4 hours and lasts for 24 hours.
Biguanides	metformin	Glucophage	Should be taken 2 to 3 times daily before meals; lasts for 12 hours.
	metformin, extended-release	Glucophage XR	Should be taken with the evening meal; lasts for 24 hours.
Combination agent	glyburide and metformin	Glucovance	Should be taken with meals; lasts for 12 hours.
Thiazolidinediones	pioglitazone rosiglitazone	Actos Avandia	These drugs should be taken once or twice a day with or without meals; peak 3 hours after ingestion and last for 16 to 34 hours.
Meglitinide	repaglinide	Prandin	Should be taken before meals; peaks in 30 to 60 minutes and lasts for 1 to 2 hours.
D-phenylalanine derivative	nateglinide	Starlix	Should be taken up to 30 minutes before each meal; peaks within 1 hour and lasts a few hours.
Alpha-glucosidase inhibitors	acarbose miglitol	Precose Glyset	Should be taken just before a meal; lasts about 1 hour.

benefit the most from the thiazolidinediones. Thiazolidinediones should be taken with food to improve absorption of the drug.

Troglitazone (Rezulin), the first drug in this class to receive FDA approval, was withdrawn from the market due to reports of rare, but severe, liver failure and related deaths. Pioglitazone and rosiglitazone are less toxic to the liver than troglitazone. Still, the FDA recommends checking liver enzymes before patients begin taking a thiazolidinedione and monitoring them regularly thereafter. Some patients with congestive heart failure may not be able

Wholesale Cost* (Generic Cost)	Comments
250 mg: $90 ($61)	Hypoglycemia is the most worrying side effect (particularly in the elderly, debilitated, or malnourished). May cause water retention, constipation, diarrhea, dizziness, headache, heartburn, increased or decreased appetite, or stomach pain/discomfort. Drinking alcohol while taking chlorpropamide can cause abdominal cramps, nausea, flushing, or headaches.
2 mg: $41 5 mg: $42 ($34)	Generally more expensive than the first-generation agent, chlorpropamide. A smaller dosage is required. Side effects are similar to those listed for chlorpropamide.
5 mg: $37	
5 mg: $74 ($65) 6 mg: $122 5 mg: $99	
500 mg: $75 500 mg: $66	May be used alone or with sulfonylureas, acarbose, or insulin. Also helps lower cholesterol and triglycerides, and may help with weight control. Does not produce hypoglycemia when used alone. May cause nausea, diarrhea, bloating, or, very rarely, a fatal buildup of lactic acid in the blood.
5 mg/500 mg: $78	See separate entries for glyburide and metformin.
15 mg: $296 4 mg: $260	May be used alone or with insulin. Side effects are uncommon, but include swelling of the hands and feet. Liver tests are advised; see text at left. Insulin dose may need to be decreased to avoid hypoglycemia. Full effects may require 2 to 8 weeks of treatment.
0.5 mg: $83	Hypoglycemia, the most frequent side effect, is less common than with sulfonylureas.
60 mg: $92	May be used alone or with metformin.
50 mg: $54 50 mg: $61	May be used alone or with sulfonylureas or metformin. May cause gas, soft stools, diarrhea, or abdominal discomfort, which tend to lessen with time.

*Average wholesale prices to pharmacists for 100 tablets of the dosage amount listed. Costs to consumers are higher. If a generic version is available, the cost is listed in parentheses. Source: *Red Book, 2001* (Medical Economics Data, publishers).

to use these drugs because they increase the volume of blood in the body, which might overtax the heart. Another possible side effect is swelling of the feet or lower legs (peripheral edema). In addition, the cholesterol-lowering medication cholestyramine (Questran) inhibits absorption of thiazolidinediones and so should not be taken at the same time of day. A major concern in people taking both a thiazolidinedione and insulin is the possible need to decrease insulin doses in order to avoid hypoglycemia, especially since the peak effect of thiazolidinediones may not occur until several weeks or even months after the drug is initiated.

The D-phenylalanine derivatives. Nateglinide (Starlix) is the newest oral blood glucose-lowering drug to be approved by the FDA (see the sidebar on the opposite page). Taken with meals, nateglinide works by stimulating rapid insulin secretion to reduce increases in blood glucose levels that occur soon after eating.

Nateglinide can be taken either by itself or in combination with metformin. The drug appears to be well tolerated, with a low risk of hypoglycemia. It seems to be most effective when post-meal glucose is unusually high, such as over 200 mg/dL. There is increasing interest in post-meal glucose among researchers, but for now it appears that good HbA1c and good pre-meal glucose control are most important.

Insulin

More than a third of patients with type 2 diabetes eventually require insulin treatment to control blood glucose levels as the severity of diabetes worsens and oral drugs lose their effectiveness. The sulfonylureas, metformin, and the thiazolidinediones are also being prescribed with increasing frequency in combination with insulin.

Types of insulin. All insulins were isolated from beef or pork pancreases until 1982, when techniques became available to produce human insulin. Only human insulin and its biosynthetic modifications are manufactured today. Three types of insulin are available: rapid-, intermediate-, and long-acting.

Regular insulin—the rapid-acting insulin—is injected 30 to 45 minutes before meals to cover the rise in blood glucose that begins about 15 minutes following food intake. An even faster-acting insulin called lispro (Humalog) was approved a few years ago by the FDA. Slightly modified from human insulin, lispro is absorbed more rapidly from injection sites and begins to work within 15 minutes of injection. Unlike conventional insulins, lispro is available only by prescription, since its effect on children and pregnant women is unknown.

Intermediate-acting insulins contain protamine (NPH insulin) or are large zinc-containing crystals of insulin (lente insulin); both substances slow the absorption of insulin from injection sites. The long-acting insulin (ultralente) has even larger zinc-insulin crystals, which further prolong the entry of insulin into the blood. Insulin glargine (Lantus), another form of modified human insulin recently approved by the FDA, provides glucose lowering over a 24-hour period. Ultralente insulin and insulin glargine are injected once or twice a day and supplemented with regular insulin before one or more meals. (For an overview of the various types of insulin, see the chart on pages 40–41.)

Typically, a combination of insulin types is used to treat diabetes. Regular or lispro insulin is often added to intermediate- or long-acting insulin before one or more meals to reduce the after-meal increase in blood glucose. For example, in the DCCT (see pages 22–24), meticulous glucose control was attained with injections of regular insulin before each meal, plus NPH or lente insulin at bedtime or ultralente insulin with the evening meal.

Regular insulin can be combined in the same syringe with intermediate- or long-acting insulin. Because the longer-acting insulins can modify the regular insulin, it is best to make the injection within five minutes after mixing the two insulin types. A notable exception is insulin glargine (Lantus), which cannot be mixed in the same syringe with other insulins.

Combining regular and NPH insulins can be simplified with the purchase of a 70/30 mixture, which contains 70% NPH and 30% regular insulin, or a 50/50 mixture, which contains 50% NPH and 50% regular insulin. The advantage of simplicity, however, is counterbalanced by the fixed ratio of the two insulins, which may not be suitable for all patients.

Modes of insulin administration. To be effective, insulin must be injected. It cannot be swallowed, because digestive enzymes would destroy the insulin before it reached the bloodstream. Injections are given subcutaneously (under the skin) at any site where there is fatty tissue. The best sites for insulin injection are detailed in the feature on page 45.

A needle and syringe are most often used for insulin injection. Other methods of injecting insulin include insulin pens, jet injectors, and external insulin pumps.

Insulin syringes. Injection with a needle and syringe—which, for years, was the only available option—remains the predominant choice for most insulin-treated patients in the United States today. Fortunately, the devices currently available—disposable, lightweight syringes, with shorter, ultrafine needles—have made daily injections more convenient and less painful than ever before.

One advantage of syringes is the wide variety of sizes and styles. Syringes may also be best for those who must mix different types of insulin into one dose; pen injectors (see below) offer less flexibility.

Insulin pens. Insulin pen injectors combine an insulin container and syringe into one compact device. Two types are available: reusable and prefilled. With reusable pens, patients load a cartridge of

NEW DRUG APPROVAL

New Oral Blood Glucose-Lowering Drug Approved for Type 2 Diabetes

The U.S. Food and Drug Administration (FDA) has approved nateglinide (Starlix), a new oral medication for treating type 2 diabetes.

Nateglinide reduces spikes in blood glucose levels after meals by stimulating the rapid production of insulin by the pancreas. It is unlike other diabetes medications since it only lowers glucose levels that rise following a meal. Metformin, for example, lowers glucose levels by improving tissue sensitivity to insulin and by decreasing glucose production in the liver.

Nateglinide is taken within 30 minutes of each meal and reaches its peak effectiveness within one hour. Its action wears off in a few hours.

In clinical trials, nateglinide reduced mean fasting blood glucose levels significantly more than a placebo. The most common side effect was low blood glucose (hypoglycemia). Rare side effects included upper respiratory infection, flu symptoms, dizziness, and joint pain.

Nateglinide should not be taken by people who have type 1 diabetes or use diabetes medications other than metformin; the drug should be used with caution in people with significant liver disease.

APPROVED BY THE FDA
December 20, 2000

Types of Insulin 2002

Type	Drug Names	Wholesale Cost*
Rapid-acting (short-acting)	*Human:*	
	Humulin R (Regular)	10 mL vial: $24
	Novolin R (Regular)	10 mL vial: $24
	Novolin R Penfill (Regular)	five 1.5 mL vials: $38
	Velosulin BR (Regular)	10 mL vial: $35
Very rapid-acting	*Modified Human:*	
	Humalog (lispro)	10 mL vial: $42
Intermediate-acting	*Human:*	
	Humulin N (NPH)	10 mL vial: $24
	Novolin N (NPH)	10 mL vial: $24
	Novolin N Penfill (NPH)	five 1.5 mL vials: $38
	Humulin L (Lente)	10 mL vial: $24
	Novolin L (Lente)	10 mL vial: $24
Long-acting	*Human:*	
	Humulin U (Ultralente)	10 mL vial: $24
	Modified Human:	
	insulin glargine (Lantus)	10 mL vial: $35
Mixtures	*Human:*	
	Humulin 50/50 (50% NPH, 50% Regular)	10 mL vial: $24
	Humulin 70/30 (70% NPH, 30% Regular)	10 mL vial: $24
	Novolin 70/30 (70% NPH, 30% Regular)	10 mL vial: $24
	Novolin 70/30 Penfill (70% NPH, 30% Regular)	five 1.5 mL vials: $38
	Novolin 70/30 Prefilled (70% NPH, 30% Regular)	five 1.5 mL vials: $40

insulin into the pen, attach a needle, and "dial in" the dose before pressing a plunger to administer the injection. The prefilled pens are easier to use than reusable pens—they contain a built-in insulin cartridge, and are discarded after the insulin is gone—but they may be more expensive.

Jet injectors. Jet injectors use a high-pressure jet of air to send a fine stream of insulin through the skin. While the elimination of needle sticks may sound appealing, these devices have had only limited use so far because they are bulky and expensive. Although they may be useful for people with an extreme fear of needles, they may be just as uncomfortable, causing pain and bruising at the injection site.

External insulin pumps. First used in the early 1980s, continuous subcutaneous insulin infusion (CSII) involves the continuous infusion of insulin by an external pump, usually worn on a belt. The in-

Onset, Peak, and Duration	Comments
Begins to work in 30 minutes to 1 hour, peaks at 2 to 4 hours, and lasts for about 6 to 8 hours.	Injected before meals to cover the sugars absorbed from food.
Begins to work in about 10 to 15 minutes, peaks at about 2 hours, and lasts for about 4 hours.	The fastest-acting insulin available.
Begins working after about 1 to 4 hours. Action peaks after about 6 to 12 hours, and effects continue for about 14 to 24 hours.	Often used in combination with rapid-acting insulin.
Action begins about 4 to 6 hours after injection; peaks after 18 to 28 hours; and lasts for up to 36 hours.	Best when combined with a rapid-acting insulin to provide proper insulin effect at mealtimes.
Varies, according to type.	Convenient for people who draw up a mixture of NPH and Regular in one syringe. Helpful for those with poor dexterity or eyesight or any persons who have problems drawing up insulin from two different bottles or reading the instructions and dosages on the bottle labels.

*Average wholesale prices to pharmacists. Costs to consumers are higher.
Source: *Red Book, 2001* (Medical Economics Data, publishers).

sulin passes through tubing (a cannula) and is delivered beneath the skin of the abdomen via a needle, which is changed by the patient every few days. The continuous insulin infusion, supplemented with additional doses of insulin through the pump with each meal, promotes excellent control of type 1 diabetes. Some people with type 2 diabetes that is hard to control may also benefit from the device.

The pumps are now small and easy to use, but this approach requires frequent daily monitoring of blood glucose, a clear understanding of diabetes and the potential dangers of failures in the CSII technique, and a stable personality. Users must be vigilant for pump malfunctions, leaks in the catheter, and inadvertent removal of the needle from its site beneath the skin. Any of these interruptions of insulin infusion can lead to a rapid fall in blood insulin levels and serious acute complications, such as ketoacidosis.

Nevertheless, CSII is highly effective for many people; it offers the possibility of improved diabetic control with the added benefit of limiting the number of needle sticks to one every two to four days. The initial unit costs about $5,000, and many, though not all, insurance companies will cover all or part of the expense. Supplies, including insulin, cost about $300 per month.

Techniques under development. Researchers are working on a variety of new approaches to insulin delivery, including inhaled insulin, nasal insulin, oral insulin, and insulin patches. Devices that allow insulin to be inhaled deep into the lungs are considered the most promising alternatives (see the sidebar on the opposite page).

Another promising means of administering insulin is an implantable insulin pump. The pump is placed under the skin in the left side of the abdomen. Insulin is delivered in small, intermittent pulses at a constant rate through the tip of a catheter that rests within the abdominal cavity. These pulses are supplemented by mealtime doses of insulin controlled via an external device that transmits commands to the pump.

The main advantages of implantable pumps appear to be tight glucose control with less hypoglycemia and less weight gain. Quality of life is improved, in part because a needle injection to refill the pump is required only every few months. The major problems with these devices have been blockage of the end of the catheter, which may require replacement of the catheter, and the need to replace the pump when the batteries wear out—after about three years. A new model is likely to last seven to eight years.

The pumps are not yet approved by the FDA. They are used only in a research setting, though the clinical trials have expanded greatly in recent years. About 1,300 people around the world have been treated with implantable pumps. Exciting progress is being made on blood glucose sensing, so that some day a "closed loop" system—in which blood glucose is automatically monitored and insulin is automatically injected—may be available.

Adverse effects of insulin. Patients taking insulin are susceptible to hypoglycemia when they administer too much insulin, delay or miss a meal, or exercise without first eating a snack. Consequently, insulin treatment requires careful attention to the timing of meals, exercise, and alcohol intake. Frequent tests of blood glucose at home, and periodic hemoglobin A1c tests by a physician, are necessary to determine the doses of insulin needed to give good control and limit bouts of hypoglycemia.

Other adverse effects of insulin are fat tissue loss (lipoatrophy) or overgrowth (lipohypertrophy) at the sites of insulin injections, allergic reactions, and insulin resistance. Alterations in fat tissue, less common with the modern insulins now available, can be further minimized by rotating injection sites. Allergic reactions, now rare, are managed by a desensitization procedure that involves injections of small amounts of insulin at first, followed by progressively larger doses. Insulin resistance, caused by the formation of antibodies against insulin or some other cause, is treated with large doses of insulin.

Treatment of Hypoglycemia

Hypoglycemia, which refers to low blood glucose, is a potential side effect of insulin, as well as of several oral drugs. There are two types of hypoglycemic symptoms: adrenergic and neurologic. Adrenergic symptoms—typically sweating, palpitations, nervousness, hunger, faintness, weakness, and numbness in the fingers and around the mouth—result when low blood glucose levels trigger the release of the hormone epinephrine into the blood. This response helps return glucose levels to normal, as does the release of glucagon from the pancreas.

These protective actions—particularly the release of glucagon—are often lost after 5 to 10 years of diabetes. Though unpleasant, adrenergic symptoms alert people with diabetes that they need to eat some sugar-containing food or drink some juice to raise their blood glucose levels rapidly. However, the symptoms of hypoglycemia may be diminished or absent in patients who are taking beta-blockers or in those who have nerve damage after many years of diabetes.

Neurologic symptoms—headache, lack of coordination, double vision, inappropriate behavior, and confusion—are a greater danger because people may become confused before they can treat themselves (and thus need another person's assistance). Extreme hypoglycemia can cause seizures, coma, or, in rare cases, permanent brain damage and death.

Certain foods and liquids are especially helpful for treating hypoglycemia. For example, 4 to 6 oz of apple or orange juice, five to seven hard candies, or glucose tablets can raise blood glucose quickly. People with diabetes should always have one of these on hand. Avoid using foods like chocolate or nuts, which do contain carbohydrates, but take longer to digest because they also contain fat. Glucagon injections can rapidly raise blood glucose levels. Some

ON THE HORIZON

Inhaled Insulin Shows Promise

Patients with diabetes who take insulin injections before meals to control their blood glucose may eventually be able to inhale the hormone instead.

A recent study evaluated inhaled insulin in 26 patients with type 2 diabetes who needed two or three insulin injections each day to regulate their blood glucose levels. The patients inhaled insulin before each meal in the form of a dry powder from a hand-held inhaler and received a bedtime injection of ultralente (long-acting) insulin.

After three months, the patients' hemoglobin A1c levels had declined from 8.67% to 7.96%, indicating a significant, though modest, improvement in blood glucose control. Inhaled insulin had no adverse effects on lung function. In addition, there were no severe hypoglycemic episodes, though 69% of the patients experienced mild to moderate hypoglycemia, which occurred more often during the first four weeks of the study.

These findings are preliminary, however. Results from the larger-scale studies that are currently underway are needed to determine whether inhaled insulin is effective and safe over the long term.

ANNALS OF INTERNAL MEDICINE
Volume 134, pages 203 and 242
February 6, 2001

people with diabetes keep glucagon in the refrigerator. Someone else can be trained to inject glucagon, in case the person with diabetes experiences a severe episode of hypoglycemia and is not alert enough to eat anything.

Pancreatic and Islet Transplants

A pancreatic transplant is considered for people with type 1 diabetes who also require a kidney transplant and whose diabetes is so difficult to control that it becomes debilitating or even life-threatening. The procedure was first developed in 1967 at the University of Minnesota, but few transplants were performed until the late 1970s. A pancreas is obtained from a deceased donor and implanted in the pelvic region. Pancreatic veins are attached to the iliac vein (which returns blood to the heart from the lower abdominal organs), allowing insulin from the transplanted organ to enter the circulatory system. About 4,000 pancreatic transplants, almost all in combination with a kidney transplant, have been performed in the last 15 years, most since 1987.

When successful, pancreatic transplants normalize blood glucose levels and thus free patients from daily insulin injections and rigid dietary control; however, there are several drawbacks to the procedure. Transplant patients must trade insulin injections for daily doses of immunosuppressive drugs, which help prevent the body from rejecting the new organ. These drugs must be taken for life and have a wide range of serious side effects, including a greater risk of infections and cancer, elevated blood pressure and blood cholesterol levels, and more rapid deterioration of kidney function.

Despite the increasing number of pancreatic transplants, it has been hard to demonstrate that a transplant can halt or reverse established diabetic complications, such as nephropathy, retinopathy, or macrovascular disease. Moreover, the failure rate is particularly high when pancreatic transplants are not done along with a kidney transplant. According to data from the International Pancreas Transplant Registry, 37% of isolated pancreatic transplants in the United States fail within a year. For this reason, the authors of a review of the current status of pancreas and kidney/pancreas transplants state that "there is at present no justification for solitary pancreas transplantation. There is one exception ... the patient whose metabolic control is so difficult that the diabetic state is itself life-threatening or incapacitating."

A combined pancreas/kidney transplant may be considered for type 1 patients who have end-stage kidney failure. This procedure

Where To Inject Insulin

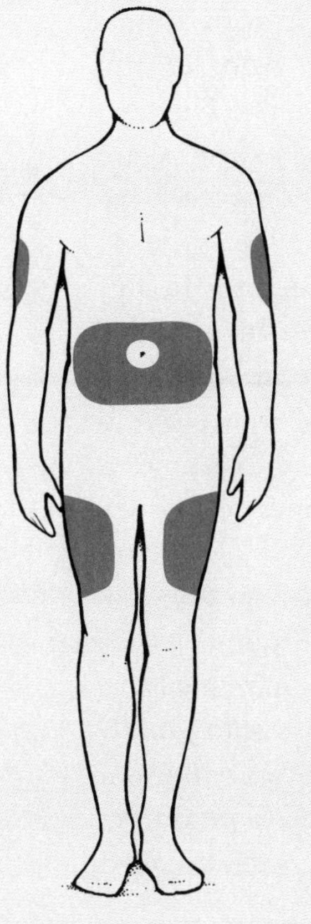

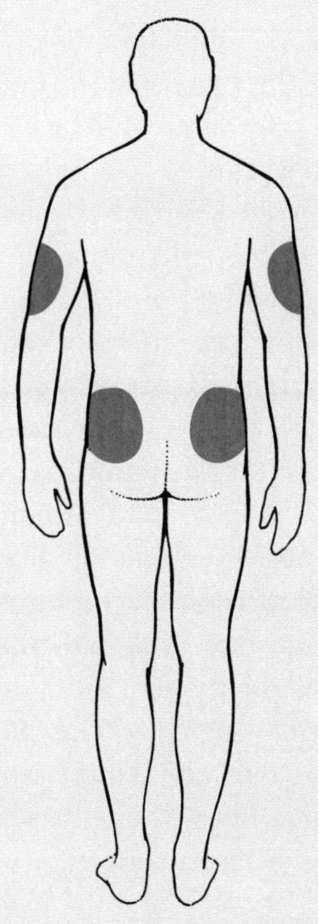

Insulin must be given by injection, since it is inactivated by digestive enzymes when taken by mouth. The daily routine of injecting insulin seems arduous at first, but most people eventually adapt to it.

The most frequently used sites for injecting insulin are the abdomen (except for a 2" area around the navel), the front and outer side of the thigh, the upper part of the buttocks, and the outer side of the upper arm (see the illustration above). Injections are given into the layer of fatty tissue under the skin. (To avoid injecting insulin into muscle, pinch a large area of skin between two fingers before inserting the needle.)

It is important to alter the location of the injections regularly either within or among the potential sites—a strategy called site rotation—because fat tissue may accumulate (lipohypertrophy) or be destroyed (lipoatrophy) if one site is used too frequently. (Lipoatrophy, however, is extremely rare today owing to improvements in the purity of insulin.) If you are using only the abdomen, for example, as an injection site, you should change the location on your abdomen from shot to shot. If you also use other sites on the body, you should rotate the sites regularly according to the time of day: for instance, you can give morning injections into the abdomen and evening injections into the thigh.

The specific site where insulin is injected affects blood glucose levels: Insulin enters the bloodstream most rapidly when injected into the abdomen, a little more slowly from the upper arms, and even more slowly from the thighs and buttocks. Thus, injecting insulin into the abdomen before breakfast and lunch will permit the insulin to be absorbed more rapidly to deal with the increase in blood glucose after a meal. Conversely, the bedtime insulin shot may be given into the thigh or buttock so that the insulin will persist longer in the bloodstream during the night.

eliminates the need for both dialysis and daily insulin injections. It is not understood why replacing both organs at the same time has a higher success rate than replacing the pancreas alone. The one-year success rate for a combined transplant is 82% in the United States, according to International Pancreas Transplant Registry data. And overall, the one-year patient survival rate in the United States is 92% for combined transplants. Another option for people with kidney failure is to have only a kidney transplant, preferably from a living donor (people can live with only one of their two kidneys). The one-year success rate for this procedure is 94%; the five-year success rate is 75%. In fact, deaths among kidney transplant patients with diabetes are mostly due to cardiovascular disease.

One drawback to a combined transplant is the need for higher doses of immunosuppressive drugs than are required after a kidney transplant alone. Patients with macrovascular disease may be ineligible for either a combined or solo kidney transplant, since blood vessel damage reduces survival rates. And, as with a solo pancreas transplant, there is no evidence that a combined pancreas/kidney transplant improves the complications of diabetes. As of yet, no studies have compared the effects of a combined transplant on diabetes complications with those of a solo pancreas transplant.

The ideal treatment may be implantation of the pancreatic islets that contain the insulin-secreting cells. This method would greatly simplify the surgery. By treating the pancreas with an enzyme that breaks up connective tissue, the islets can be separated from the remaining pancreatic tissue. Isolated human islets have been placed in the kidney, the abdominal cavity, and the liver.

This approach has been hampered by difficulties in obtaining the large number of human islets needed to secrete enough insulin, and by the rapid decline in function of implanted islets, possibly due to damage by the immunosuppressive drugs required to prevent their rejection. One way to overcome these problems might be to produce insulin-secreting cells from stem cells.

A number of ingenious approaches to transplanting islets are in development. One method was tested by a group of researchers from Canada. They transplanted large numbers of pancreatic islets into the livers of seven patients with type 1 diabetes, using a combination of new immunosuppressive drugs that do not contain steroids. One year after the transplant, all seven patients were able to control blood glucose without the need for insulin injections. Studies on this technique are being conducted at a number of medical centers. Although promising, this approach is still experimental.

Alternative Treatments

In recent years, a growing interest and market has emerged for the use of "alternative" therapies to manage diabetes. Several natural remedies and nutritional supplements—including chromium, *gymnea sylvestre,* and vanadium—reportedly reduce blood glucose levels; others—for example, alpha-lipoic acid, evening primrose oil, ginkgo biloba, and chelation therapy—purport to treat or prevent the major complications of diabetes.

There is little or no hard medical evidence that any of these alternatives are as effective as insulin or oral diabetes drugs in controlling blood glucose or preventing complications. Patients wishing to try one of these options should do so in addition to, not instead of, their prescribed treatment regimen. And they should do so only with their doctor's knowledge.

TREATMENT OF DIABETIC COMPLICATIONS

If diabetic complications develop, they must be treated along with the diabetes itself.

Retinopathy

Laser photocoagulation halts or retards the decline in vision from diabetic retinopathy in most patients, if it is carried out before too much damage has occurred. The procedure is done on an outpatient basis, often over several visits. The ophthalmologist dilates the pupil with eye drops and then targets a series of spots on the retina with a sharp burst of laser light, causing tiny scars to form. The procedure prevents the small vessels from rupturing and bleeding into the vitreous humor.

Laser treatment reduces the chance of blindness by half in those with proliferative retinopathy. Though extensive photocoagulation usually diminishes peripheral vision and may decrease night vision, its success in preserving visual acuity makes it worthwhile despite these side effects. Laser treatment also helps preserve vision when used to treat what is called "clinically significant macular edema." Only a qualified ophthalmologist can determine when laser treatment is needed.

If the extent or location of the damage makes photocoagulation ineffective, or if the vitreous humor is too clouded with blood, vision may be improved with a vitrectomy, a surgical procedure that removes the vitreous humor and replaces it with a saline solution. Roughly 70% of people who have vitrectomies notice an improvement or stabilization of their sight, and some recover enough vision to resume reading as well as driving.

Because photocoagulation works so remarkably well if done in

NEW RESEARCH

Drug May Reduce CHD Risk In People With Diabetes

The medication fenofibrate (Tricor), primarily used to lower blood triglyceride levels, may reduce the risk of coronary heart disease (CHD) events in people with diabetes, a new study finds.

Researchers randomized 418 people with type 2 diabetes to receive either 200 mg of fenofibrate or a placebo daily for three years. Blood lipid levels were measured every four months, and an angiogram to visualize coronary arteries was performed at the beginning and end of the study.

The fenofibrate group showed significant decreases in levels of total cholesterol, LDL cholesterol, and triglycerides compared with the placebo group. HDL cholesterol, which protects against CHD, increased significantly more in the fenofibrate group, as well. Angiogram results revealed that markers of CHD progression were reduced in the fenofibrate group. During the study and the subsequent six months, the fenofibrate group experienced fewer heart attacks and required fewer CHD-related medical procedures, although the differences were not statistically significant.

The authors conclude that correcting abnormal blood lipid levels is important for preventing the progression of CHD in people with diabetes. They recommend that blood lipid levels be measured at the time diabetes is diagnosed and annually thereafter.

THE LANCET
Volume 357, page 905
March 24, 2001

time, and because even advanced retinopathy can be asymptomatic, it is crucial for people with type 2 diabetes to begin seeing their ophthalmologist for annual eye examinations when their diabetes is first diagnosed. For people with type 1 diabetes, annual eye examinations should start no later than five years after diagnosis.

Nephropathy

Four strategies are used to prevent nephropathy or slow its progression. Tight glucose control is one method (see pages 22–24). Treating high blood pressure, common in diabetes, is extremely important. High blood pressure damages the kidneys, which in turn raises blood pressure further. Restricting dietary protein is another way to delay the course of kidney disease. The fourth and most recent strategy is treatment with angiotensin-converting enzyme (ACE) inhibitors, a class of drugs commonly prescribed to treat high blood pressure. (These strategies are discussed in more detail in the feature on pages 50–51.)

ACE inhibitors such as captopril (Capoten) and enalapril (Vasotec) are particularly effective in slowing the progression of kidney disease to kidney failure. This benefit is independent of the effects of ACE inhibitors on blood pressure. ACE inhibitors work by slowing the production of the hormone angiotensin, which elevates the pressure across the walls of the small blood vessels in the glomeruli, the sites of blood filtration in the kidneys. Researchers believe that even in the absence of high blood pressure, an abnormally high pressure in the glomeruli of people with diabetes can gradually destroy the vessels in the kidney.

Other blood pressure drugs such as the angiotensin II receptor blockers irbesartan (Avapro) and losartan (Cozaar), which prevent the actions of angiotensin by inhibiting it from binding to its tissue receptors, have also been shown to slow the progression of kidney disease in people with diabetes (see the sidebars on the opposite page and page 53). Similar to the ACE inhibitors, the benefit of these drugs is independent of their blood pressuring-lowering effects.

Once kidney failure occurs, treatment is directed toward slowing the accumulation of waste products in the blood. Limitation of protein intake is necessary to decrease a buildup of the breakdown products of ingested proteins; at the same time the diet must contain enough protein to prevent malnutrition. Antacids, such as aluminum hydroxide, are given to bind dietary phosphate in the intestine. This prevents marked increases in levels of blood phosphate that can, in turn, lower blood calcium levels. Calcium supplements may be necessary to raise blood calcium levels and prevent injury to the bones. Tablets containing sodium bicarbonate are often needed to counteract the acidic condition of the blood in kidney failure.

Anemia, with associated weakness and fatigue, invariably accompanies chronic kidney failure; it can be improved with the use of erythropoietin, a hormone that stimulates the production of red blood cells. Many common medications are normally excreted by the kidneys. In kidney failure, the doses of such drugs must be decreased to avoid their buildup to toxic levels. Kidney dialysis is usually initiated when kidney function deteriorates to less than 10% of normal—a condition called end-stage kidney disease.

Neuropathy

It is often difficult to treat symptoms that result from diabetic neuropathy. Improved control of blood glucose levels is the first step in treatment.

Amitriptyline (Amitid, Amitril, Elavil, Emitrip, Endep, Enovil, Vanatrip), usually used as an antidepressant drug, is often the most effective medication for relieving the symptoms of symmetrical peripheral neuropathy; the medication works in much the same way as it does to relieve depression—by making more norepinephrine available to nerve cells. (Norepinephrine is a neurotransmitter, a chemical that carries messages between nerve cells.) However, in some people, amitriptyline produces troublesome side effects—drowsiness, urinary retention (the inability to empty the bladder completely), and a severe drop in blood pressure upon standing. These effects can be minimized by taking the drug at bedtime, as well as by starting with a small dose that is gradually increased. One study found that desipramine (Norpramin), another antidepressant, can be almost as effective and has fewer adverse effects.

Gabapentin (Neurontin) is another option, either alone or in combination with amitriptyline. An anticonvulsant approved for epilepsy in 1994, gabapentin is generally well tolerated. When side effects (typically drowsiness and confusion) occur, they usually can be minimized by adjusting the dosage. According to recently published studies, gabapentin should be considered for peripheral neuropathy when antidepressant drugs fail or produce significant side effects.

The symptoms of autonomic neuropathy, which include stomach and bowel problems and sexual dysfunction, can also be alleviated. Treatment of these and other symptoms of autonomic neuropathy are discussed in the feature on pages 14–15.

NEW RESEARCH

Irbesartan Helps Prevent Kidney Disease in People With Diabetes

The antihypertensive drug irbesartan can help prevent or delay the progression of kidney damage in people with hypertension (high blood pressure) and type 2 diabetes, two recent studies show.

One study evaluated irbesartan in 1,715 hypertensive patients with kidney damage due to type 2 diabetes. The participants were given irbesartan (Avapro, 300 mg/day), another antihypertensive drug called amlodipine (Norvasc, 10 mg/day), or a placebo.

Patients treated with irbesartan were significantly less likely to experience a doubling of their blood creatinine level (a sign of declining kidney function) than those in the other study groups. In addition, the risk of end-stage kidney disease was 23% lower in patients treated with irbesartan than in either of the other groups.

The second study was conducted in 590 hypertensive patients with type 2 diabetes who had microalbuminuria (small amounts of protein in the urine) but no other evidence of kidney disease. Two doses of irbesartan (150 mg/day and 300 mg/day) were compared with a placebo. After two years, the higher dose of irbesartan had significantly reduced the development of overt kidney disease.

Irbesartan may act similarly to ACE inhibitors, which also protect against progression of kidney disease in people with diabetes.

THE NEW ENGLAND JOURNAL OF MEDICINE
Volume 345, pages 851 and 870
September 20, 2001

Preserving Kidney Function When You Have Diabetes

Nephropathy, or kidney damage, is a potential long-term complication of diabetes. It can result in kidney failure, which can only be treated with dialysis or a kidney transplant. Fortunately, most people with diabetes do not develop kidney problems, and several steps can be taken to prevent kidney damage or halt its progression.

Kidney Function and Dysfunction
The kidneys filter waste and excess fluid from the blood. Blood enters the kidney through an artery and then passes through the glomeruli—clusters of capillaries that act as filters. After filtration, the cleaned blood, along with its essential proteins, returns to the rest of the body through a vein, while waste products and excess fluid pass into the urine. (See the illustration at right.)

In people with diabetes, high blood glucose and high blood pressure can damage the glomeruli and allow protein to leak into the urine. In the early stages of kidney damage (usually 10 to 15 years after the onset of diabetes), the small amount of protein that leaks into the urine is called microalbuminuria. As damage progresses, the kidneys are not as effective at removing waste products. The result is an accumulation of waste products in the blood and more protein in the urine. (This is referred to as proteinuria.) If the kidney damage becomes worse, the kidneys may eventually fail.

Kidney damage cannot be reversed once it occurs, and its effects are usually not felt until the damage is severe. Therefore, you should take measures early in the course of diabetes to prevent kidney damage or stop its progress.

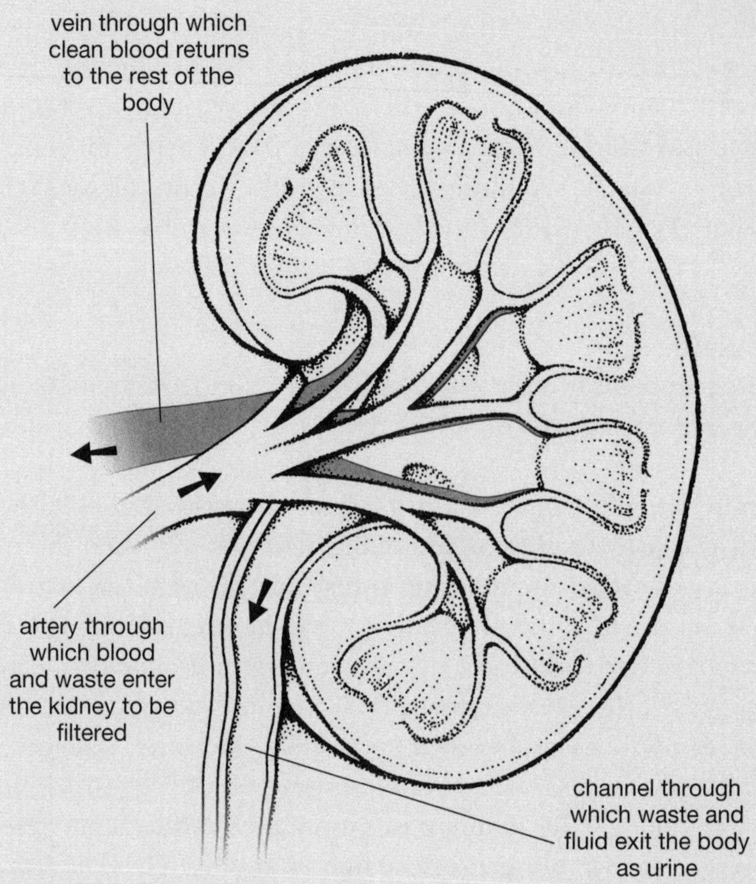

Evaluating Your Risk
Because people from certain ethnic groups are at greater risk for developing diabetic nephropathy, these individuals should take extra care to protect their kidneys. Between 40% and 50% of Native Americans with diabetes will develop kidney damage; so will 20% to 30% of Hispanic and black people with diabetes. In comparison, about 10% of whites with diabetes will develop kidney damage.

Diabetic Foot Problems

Because people with diabetes often develop poor circulation in the extremities due to atherosclerosis, they are especially vulnerable to infections and gangrene in their feet. At the same time, nerve damage from diabetes can diminish the normal warning signs of foot pain so that infections and injuries go unnoticed. One fifth of hospitalizations for diabetes are due to foot infections, and 86,000 amputations are performed each year because of diabetic complications.

Having a first-degree relative (a parent or sibling) with diabetic nephropathy also increases your risk. Furthermore, men with diabetes have a 50% greater chance of developing kidney problems than women with diabetes. However, if you have lived with diabetes for more than 40 years without any kidney disease, you most likely will never develop such problems.

Preventing Kidney Failure Or Halting Its Progression

According to the American Diabetes Association, everyone with diabetes should be tested regularly for microalbuminuria. People with type 1 diabetes should receive this test first in puberty, then five years after the diagnosis, and every year after that. For people with type 2 diabetes, testing should take place at the time of diagnosis and yearly thereafter. Ask your doctor if you need other tests for kidney damage, such as those that measure creatinine and urea in the blood. Early detection should stimulate aggressive measures to prevent kidney failure.

To prevent kidney problems, or to halt their progression if tests show you have microalbuminuria or proteinuria, you should take the following measures. First, be sure to maintain tight blood glucose control. If you develop microalbuminuria you are at increased risk for proteinuria, but you can cut this risk in half by maintaining good control of your glucose levels. Second, maintain or reduce your blood pressure. According to the National Kidney Foundation, people with diabetes should maintain a blood pressure of 130/80 mm Hg or lower. To do so, you may have to lose weight, exercise, consume less sodium, limit alcohol, and stop smoking.

In most cases, medications are also needed to lower blood pressure. At least 65% of people with diabetes and high blood pressure will need more than one medication to bring their blood pressure under control, according to the National Kidney Foundation. ACE inhibitors (see pages 48 and 53) should be used first. Most people with diabetes who test positive for microalbuminuria or proteinuria should take an ACE inhibitor no matter what their blood pressure. Patients may need a diuretic along with an ACE inhibitor to reduce blood pressure further.

If you cannot achieve a blood pressure of 130/80 mm Hg with an ACE inhibitor and a diuretic, your doctor may add another drug called a calcium channel blocker. If you still have not reached the target blood pressure, your doctor may also prescribe a beta-blocker or an alpha/beta-blocker (if your resting heart rate is 84 beats per minute or more) or another type of calcium channel blocker (if your resting heart rate is below 84). A few patients may require further treatment.

Third, you should work out a diet plan with your doctor or dietitian and follow this plan closely to prevent kidney damage or slow its progression. You may be asked to eat less protein and sodium. Although it has not been proven, large amounts of protein may cause the kidneys to work harder and accelerate kidney dysfunction. The American Diabetes Association recommends that 10% to 20% of your calories come from protein, and lower levels may be appropriate when kidney damage is present.

Furthermore, do not overuse pain medications, such as aspirin, acetaminophen (Tylenol), or ibuprofen (Advil). These drugs can all exacerbate existing kidney disease or raise the risk that a person with diabetes will develop kidney damage. Taking low-dose aspirin to protect against heart disease is not a problem, but talk to your doctor about the correct dose.

Be sure to treat immediately any bladder or kidney infection that you may develop. Symptoms of these infections include a burning sensation while urinating, a frequent urge to urinate, reddish or cloudy urine, a shaky feeling, fever, or pain in your back or on your side below the ribs.

Last, the contrast agents used for some imaging tests may worsen kidney damage. To prevent this from happening, your doctor may tell you to drink plenty of water before and after the test, or will choose a test that does not require a contrast agent.

Yet proper foot care can eliminate or greatly reduce these risks.

Everyone with diabetes, but especially those with established neuropathy or poor circulation, should make a routine of good foot care. This routine involves inspecting each foot daily and carefully treating and monitoring even the most trivial cut or abrasion. When they occur, abrasions should be washed with warm water and soap, cleaned with a mild antiseptic (for example, Bactine), and then covered with a dry, sterile dressing and paper tape. Ulcers are extremely serious and must be brought to the attention of a doctor immediately. Toenails should be neatly trimmed, cut straight across rather than rounded at the ends. And at least twice a year, each foot should be examined by a physician or podiatrist. The following are some additional foot-care suggestions.

Do the following:

- Bathe feet daily in warm, soapy water and pat them dry.
- Keep feet warm and dry. Wear warm socks in the winter; keep feet cool in the summer.
- Take off shoes and put feet up from time to time during the day.
- Get regular exercise: It will help keep feet in good condition and may improve circulation somewhat.
- Tell the doctor of any unusual feelings of cold, numbness, tingling, burning, or fatigue in the feet or legs.

Do not do the following:

- Put hot-water bottles or electric heating pads on the feet—they may cause unnoticed burns.
- Sit with legs crossed, or expose feet and legs to cold or heat (for example, prolonged exposure to sunlight).
- Soak the feet—unless recommended by a doctor.
- Wear garters or tight-fitting socks, stockings, or shoes.
- Smoke—smoking reduces circulation to the feet.
- Put off seeing a physician or podiatrist if any problems develop, however minor.

Macrovascular Disease

With few exceptions, preventive measures and treatment of macrovascular disease are the same in people with diabetes as in others. High levels of blood cholesterol and high blood pressure—major risk factors for macrovascular disease—are initially treated with diet and lifestyle modifications in an effort to bring these conditions under control without medication. In fact, many of these lifestyle measures—such as a low-fat, high-carbohydrate diet, weight loss, and exercise—are the same as the ones recommended by the ADA for patients with diabetes. Medication is generally needed if elevated cholesterol or blood pressure persists despite strict adherence to these measures. Targets are less than 100 mg/dL for LDL cholesterol and less than 130/85 mm Hg for blood pressure.

To lower blood cholesterol in diabetic patients, HMG-CoA reductase inhibitors (statins) or bile acid sequestrants are often prescribed, since these drugs effectively reduce total and LDL cholesterol levels. The statins include atorvastatin (Lipitor), fluvastatin (Lescol), lovastatin (Mevacor), pravastatin (Pravachol), and simvastatin (Zocor). Cerivastatin (Baycol) was taken off the market in 2001 after it was found to be linked to fatal muscle problems. The bile acid sequestrants are cholestyramine (Questran), colesevelam (Welchol), and colestipol (Colestid).

The statins are usually the drug of choice because they are more effective and easier to take than bile acid sequestrants. Two large studies have shown a significant reduction in all cardiovascular events when patients with diabetes and known CHD had their cholesterol levels lowered with one of the statins. Nicotinic acid (niacin) is less often recommended for people with diabetes because it can elevate blood glucose levels, but it is the most effective medication to raise HDL cholesterol levels.

Triglyceride levels above 300 mg/dL—common in diabetes—are most effectively treated with gemfibrozil (Lopid) or fenofibrate (Tricor). More modest elevations in triglycerides may be treated successfully with one of the HMG-CoA reductase inhibitors, which do not lower triglyceride levels as much as gemfibrozil or fenofibrate, but are far more effective in reducing total and LDL cholesterol.

There are four classes of commonly used antihypertensive drugs: diuretics, beta-blockers, ACE inhibitors, and calcium channel blockers. Which drug is prescribed depends on many factors, such as cost or possible adverse reactions to a class of drugs. An ACE inhibitor is generally considered the preferred drug in people with diabetes because it can both lower blood pressure and help protect the kidneys from nephropathy. The Heart Outcomes Prevention Evaluation (HOPE) study showed that treatment with the ACE inhibitor ramipril (Altace) significantly reduced the number of cardiovascular complications over a five-year period in people with diabetes and one other risk factor for CHD, as well as in nondiabetics with known CHD. A surprising finding was that ramipril also decreased the occurrence of new diabetes by about 30% (see the sidebar on page 21).

Diuretics, however, may raise blood glucose levels, and beta-blockers are used with caution—especially in those treated with insulin—because they may block the warning symptoms of hypoglycemia. Beta-blockers work by impeding the action of epinephrine, the hormone responsible for producing the sweating, nervousness, and hunger that forewarn people of hypoglycemia. In the absence

NEW RESEARCH

Losartan Protects Kidney Function in Type 2 Diabetes

The antihypertensive drug losartan (Cozaar) can slow the progression of kidney disease in patients with type 2 diabetes and kidney damage, according to a recent study.

The study involved 1,513 patients who had type 2 diabetes and kidney damage; more than 96% also had high blood pressure. The patients received losartan (either 50 or 100 mg once daily) or a placebo. About 94% of the patients were also being treated with other antihypertensive medications.

During an average follow-up period of 3.4 years, the investigators found that losartan significantly preserved kidney function. Compared with the placebo, losartan reduced the doubling of serum creatinine level (a measure of declining kidney function) by 25% and lowered the risk of end-stage kidney disease by 28%. The beneficial effects of losartan on kidney function could not be explained entirely by its blood pressure-lowering effects.

Based on the reduction in end-stage kidney disease, the authors estimate that losartan in combination with conventional antihypertensive therapy could delay the need for kidney dialysis or transplantation by about two years in people with type 2 diabetes and kidney disease.

THE NEW ENGLAND JOURNAL OF MEDICINE
Volume 345, pages 861 and 910
September 20, 2001

of these symptoms, blood glucose could fall to dangerously low levels without the person being aware of it.

Diabetes produces changes in the blood that make it more prone to clotting, thus increasing the risk of a heart attack. Aspirin, which reduces the tendency of the blood to clot, has been shown to lower the incidence of heart attacks in people with or without known heart disease. In fact, an Israeli study found that taking aspirin decreased the death rate from heart disease and other causes in people with diabetes and CHD even more than in people who had CHD but not diabetes. Daily doses ranging from 80 to 325 mg (one baby aspirin or one adult aspirin daily) are effective.

Angina—chest pain due to the reduction of blood flow to the heart—can be treated with drugs or surgery. Most often angina is precipitated by restricted blood flow resulting from the buildup of plaques in the coronary arteries. Nitrates—such as nitroglycerin—can alleviate angina when it occurs. Nitroglycerin can also be used prophylactically when engaging in activities that are likely to cause chest pain, such as walking or playing tennis. Long-acting nitrates or nitroglycerin patches often help to prevent angina.

Coronary artery bypass surgery and percutaneous transluminal coronary angioplasty are surgical treatments for angina. In bypass surgery, an internal mammary artery (which usually supplies blood to the chest wall) is redirected to a site beyond the narrowed portion of a coronary artery or, less preferably, a portion of a vein from the leg is surgically attached on both sides of the blockage(s). In either case, blood flow is rerouted through the new vessel, which passes around the narrowed segment of artery.

In angioplasty, a catheter with a balloon at its tip is inserted into the femoral artery in the groin and guided to the coronary arteries in the heart. Once the catheter is positioned inside the narrowed portion of the artery, the cardiologist inflates the balloon several times to squeeze the plaque against the wall of the artery, thus widening the arterial opening and increasing blood flow to the heart. (In most angioplasty procedures, a metal tube, called a stent, is implanted in the artery to keep it propped open.)

The choice between bypass surgery and angioplasty depends on many factors, including the extent of CHD and the location of the blockage. Recent studies have shown an advantage for bypass surgery in those diabetes patients who can withstand this more invasive procedure (which requires a longer recovery period than angioplasty). One ongoing study of 1,829 patients found that for people with diabetes, survival at seven years was significantly better

Therapeutic Shoes for People With Diabetes

Roughly two thirds of people with diabetes eventually develop some degree of nerve damage. The most common type of nerve damage is peripheral neuropathy, which produces a gradual loss of sensation in the limbs, especially in the feet and lower legs. As a result, these people are less able to notice injuries that can lead to skin ulcers, particularly on the foot. Poor circulation to the legs, which is also present in some people with diabetes, impairs healing of even small wounds, leaving feet susceptible to infections and subsequent gangrene. Further, as diabetes progresses, some people may lose the natural fat pad that protects the foot.

Well-cushioned athletic or walking shoes provide adequate foot protection for many people with diabetes. However, people with reduced sensation in their feet, a history of foot ulcers, or foot deformities may require therapeutic footwear, which can reduce the chances of experiencing a break in the skin that could lead to nonhealing ulcers and even amputation.

The objective of therapeutic footwear is to protect the feet by distributing the pressure exerted by a person's weight across a larger section of the sole of the foot. This reduces the chance that excessive pressure on any one point of the sole will lead to a break in the skin.

There are various types of therapeutic footwear for people with diabetes. People with a loss of sensation in their feet may benefit from a soft insert placed in the shoe. Though not custom fitted, such inserts mold to the foot's shape through the constant force of the body's weight. They provide an extra cushion and relieve pressure on the sole of the foot. These inserts need to be modified or replaced every six months (or sooner) and may require wearing a depth shoe because of the insert's thickness. (A depth shoe looks like a walking or athletic shoe but has more room to accommodate inserts or differently-shaped feet.)

People with significant foot deformity and a loss of foot sensation often find that custom-molded inserts (called orthoses) are most beneficial. Those with a history of ulcers on the bottom of their feet often require custom-fitted shoes, which are designed from a mold of the person's feet. People with a loss of sensation, deformities, and a history of ulcers may need custom-fitted shoes and orthoses.

Despite these needs, only about 15% of people with diabetes wear orthoses and only around 12% wear therapeutic shoes. Furthermore, less than 8% of people with diabetes have their therapeutic orthoses or footwear paid for by Medicare or private insurance. In fact, many people do not know that Medicare pays for up to 80% of the cost of therapeutic footwear for certain people.

Passed in 1993, the Medicare Therapeutic Shoe Bill applies to people covered under Medicare Part B insurance. To qualify for partial reimbursement under the bill, a person must have diabetes and current or past foot complications related to neuropathy or poor circulation. Also, the person must be receiving treatment for diabetes and need therapeutic footwear because of the disease.

Each year, Medicare will cover three sets of inserts or orthoses and one pair of depth shoes or custom-fitted shoes. Shoe modification is also covered, but only in place of a pair of inserts or orthoses.

For patients to receive coverage, the doctor (either a medical doctor or a doctor of osteopathy) who is treating the patient for diabetes must complete a "Certification Statement for Therapeutic Footwear." Typically, a second doctor (a medical doctor, podiatrist, or orthopedic foot surgeon) will then prescribe the footwear by filling out a "Prescription Form for Therapeutic Footwear." The patient can then have the prescription filled by an orthotist, podiatrist, prosthetist, or pedorthist (a specialist who evaluates and designs orthoses and shoes).

Although the bill covered 1.25 million pairs of shoes in 2000, the program is underutilized. Ask your doctor if you qualify.

with bypass surgery (76%) than with angioplasty (56%).

Immediately after a heart attack, people with diabetes may be able to lower their mortality rate by regularly taking insulin. In a recent study of heart attack survivors (most had type 2 diabetes), one group of patients was brought to normal blood glucose levels with infusions of insulin and glucose in the hospital. The patients then gave themselves insulin injections four times a day for at least three months. Another group received conventional care for their diabetes. After a year, the overall mortality rate in the intensive treatment group was 19%, compared with 26% in the other group—a 29% reduction.

A review of studies found that people with diabetes also benefit from beta-blockers and ACE inhibitors after a heart attack. Beta-blockers given promptly after a heart attack reduced mortality by 37% in patients with diabetes vs. 13% in nondiabetics; long-term treatment reduced mortality by 48% in diabetic patients vs. 33% in nondiabetics. ACE inhibitors, especially given within 24 to 36 hours of a heart attack, had similar results. One study found that taking ACE inhibitors within 36 hours of a heart attack reduced mortality by up to 44% in patients with type 1 diabetes and 24.5% in those with type 2 diabetes. ■

GLOSSARY

adrenergic symptoms—Symptoms, including sweating and palpitations, that occur when a low blood glucose level triggers the release of the hormone epinephrine (adrenaline) into the blood.

alpha-glucosidase inhibitors—Oral diabetes drugs that lower the peak levels of blood glucose and insulin after a meal. They act by inhibiting intestinal enzymes that digest complex carbohydrates and sucrose, and thus delay the absorption of carbohydrates. Examples are acarbose (Precose) and miglitol (Glyset).

angiotensin-converting enzyme (ACE) inhibitors—Commonly prescribed to treat high blood pressure, this class of drugs also slows the progression of kidney disease in people with diabetes.

antioxidants—Substances that help the body neutralize free radicals, which can cause cell damage. Naturally occurring antioxidants include beta carotene, vitamin C, and vitamin E.

atherosclerosis—An accumulation of deposits of fat and fibrous tissue, called plaques, within the walls of arteries that can narrow vessels and reduce blood flow.

autonomic neuropathy—Damage to nerves that control many involuntary actions in the body, such as the movement of food through the digestive tract, heart rate, and bladder control.

biguanides—Oral diabetes drugs that enhance the action of insulin to decrease glucose production by the liver and to increase glucose uptake by muscle and fat cells. Do not cause hypoglycemia when used alone. Metformin (Glucophage) is the only available biguanide.

blood osmolarity—The thickness of the blood. High blood glucose increases blood osmolarity, making a person thirsty.

cataract—A cloudiness or opacification of the lens of the eye that can lead to visual impairment.

diabetic foot ulcer—An open sore on the foot that occurs in people with diabetes who have damage to nerves and/or poor blood flow to the feet.

diabetic ketoacidosis—An acute complication of diabetes, usually type 1, resulting from a nearly complete lack of insulin. The body is forced to use fatty acids instead of glucose as a major source of energy. The resulting excessive breakdown of fatty acids to ketone bodies raises the acidity of the blood to dangerous levels. Symptoms include nausea, vomiting, heavy breathing, and the symptoms of elevated blood glucose.

diuretics—Drugs that increase urine production by enhancing loss of sodium through the kidneys. They are used to eliminate excess fluid from the body and to treat high blood pressure.

D-phenylalanine derivatives—Oral diabetes drugs that stimulate rapid insulin secretion to reduce the rise in blood glucose levels that occurs soon after eating. The only available example is nateglinide (Starlix).

external insulin pump—A pump, usually worn on a belt, that delivers a continuous flow of insulin along with added amounts at mealtime through a plastic insert or needle inserted under the skin of the abdomen.

free radicals—Chemical compounds that can damage cells and oxidize low density lipoproteins, making them more likely to deposit in the walls of arteries.

fructosamine test—A test that measures protein-bound glucose and reflects average blood glucose levels over the prior two weeks. Similar to the more commonly performed hemoglobin A1c test but less well standardized.

gestational diabetes—A type of diabetes that occurs first during pregnancy. It occurs in 2% to 5% of pregnant women, usually goes away when the pregnancy is over, and signals a high risk of developing type 2 diabetes later in life.

glaucoma—An eye disease characterized by increased pressure within the eyeball and damage to the optic nerve.

glucagon—A hormone that raises blood glucose levels by signaling the liver to convert amino acids and glycogen to glucose and to send the glucose into the bloodstream. Glucagon may be given by injection to raise blood glucose levels in the case of a severe insulin reaction.

glucose—A simple sugar that circulates in the blood and provides energy to the body. Excess glucose is normally converted to glycogen or triglycerides, mainly in the liver, when there is adequate insulin in the blood.

glucose transport proteins—Proteins that carry glucose from the outside of a cell to the inside.

glycogen—A complex carbohydrate that is stored in the liver and muscles until it is needed for energy.

hemoglobin A1c (HbA1c) test—A test that measures the amount of glucose attached to hemoglobin. The test is routinely used to assess blood glucose control over the previous two to three months. Also called a glycohemoglobin test.

HMG-CoA reductase inhibitors—Drugs that reduce blood levels of cholesterol by blocking its formation. Also called statins.

human insulin—Insulin made by recombinant DNA procedures for use by people with diabetes. Available in various durations of action (rapid-, intermediate-, and long-acting).

hyperglycemia—High blood glucose levels.

hyperinsulinemia—Excess insulin in the blood.

GLOSSARY—continued

hyperosmolar nonketotic state—A medical emergency characterized by extremely high blood glucose levels in people with type 2 diabetes. It is usually caused by the stress of an injury or a major illness accompanied by extreme dehydration.

hypoglycemia—Low blood glucose levels. May be symptomless or may cause symptoms like shaking and sweating. May progress to changes in mental status (confusion, sleepiness) or even coma. Almost always reversed by eating carbohydrates or, if necessary, by injecting glucagon or glucose.

impaired fasting glucose—A condition in which fasting blood glucose levels are above normal (110 to 125 mg/dL) but not quite in the diabetic range.

impaired glucose tolerance—A condition in which the results of a glucose tolerance test are above normal (between 140 and 199 mg/dL two hours after ingesting 75 g of glucose) but not quite in the diabetic range.

implantable insulin pump—A pump, placed under the skin of the abdomen, that delivers insulin through a catheter into the abdominal cavity at a constant rate, along with added amounts for meals. The device is still under development and is not yet approved by the U.S. Food and Drug Administration.

insulin—A hormone normally produced by the pancreas that regulates the production of glucose by the liver and the utilization of glucose by muscle cells. Without adequate insulin, glucose accumulates in the blood and causes hyperglycemia, the hallmark of diabetes. Insulin may be taken as a medication by people with diabetes whose pancreas does not make enough insulin.

insulin pen—A combined insulin container and needle that makes injection of insulin more convenient.

insulin resistance syndrome—A group of findings, including elevated blood insulin levels, high triglycerides, low HDL cholesterol, increased risk of diabetes and atherosclerosis, and high blood pressure, that is caused by a genetic predisposition to insulin resistance and an accumulation of fat in the abdomen. Also called syndrome X or metabolic syndrome.

insulin syringe—A syringe with a needle that is used to inject insulin. The number of units of insulin are noted on the syringe.

intermediate-acting insulin—Insulin medication that begins working in 1 to 4 hours, peaks at 6 to 12 hours, and lasts for about 14 to 24 hours. Examples are NPH insulin and lente insulin.

jet injector—A needle-free way of injecting insulin that uses a high-pressure jet of air to send a fine stream of insulin through the skin.

long-acting insulin—Insulin medication that begins working in 4 to 6 hours, peaks at 18 to 28 hours, and lasts for up to 36 hours. Examples are glargine (Lantus) and ultralente insulin.

macular edema—A swelling of the macula, a small area at the center of the retina of the eye that is responsible for central and fine-detail vision. Swelling is caused by leakage and accumulation of fluid.

meglitinides—Oral diabetes drugs that induce the secretion of insulin by the pancreas in a way that is dependent on the amount of glucose in the blood. These drugs have a more rapid effect on insulin levels than sulfonylureas. The first drug in this class is repaglinide (Prandin).

metabolic syndrome—See **insulin resistance syndrome**.

mononeuropathy—Nerve damage resulting from disruption of the blood supply to one nerve. Leads to the sudden onset of pain or weakness in the area served by the affected nerve.

necrobiosis lipoidica diabeticorum (NLD)—A complication of diabetes characterized by a violet-colored area of thinned skin, an inch or more in diameter, on the front of the lower leg.

nephropathy—Kidney damage that can lead to kidney failure.

neuropathy—Nerve damage due to diabetes. Most often affects the toes or feet, and can also cause erectile dysfunction.

oral glucose tolerance test—A test in which a person fasts overnight and then drinks a solution containing 75 g of glucose. A diabetes diagnosis is made if two hours later the blood glucose level is 200 mg/dL or more.

pancreas—An organ, located behind and beneath the lower part of the stomach, that produces and secretes insulin. The pancreas also makes digestive juices.

pancreatic islets—Cellular masses in the pancreas that contain insulin-secreting cells.

peripheral neuropathy—A slow, progressive loss of function of the sensory nerves in the limbs that causes numbness, tingling, and pain in the legs and hands.

peripheral vascular disease—A buildup of fatty deposits and fibrous tissue, called plaques, in the arteries leading to the legs and feet.

photocoagulation—A laser treatment for retinopathy that slows the progression of proliferative retinopathy by destroying the small new blood vessels on the retina.

rapid-acting insulin—Insulin medication that begins working in 30 minutes to an hour, peaks at 2 to 4 hours, and lasts for about 6 to 8 hours. Examples are regular insulin and lispro (Humalog).

retinopathy—Damage to the retina caused by changes in the tiny blood vessels that supply the retina. Advanced disease may require treatment with a procedure called photocoagulation.

sulfonylureas—Oral diabetes drugs that stimulate the pancreas to secrete more insulin. Examples are chlorpropamide (Diabinese) and glyburide (DiaBeta, Glynase, Micronase).

syndrome X—See **insulin resistance syndrome**.

thiazolidinediones—Oral diabetes drugs that increase the sensitivity of muscle cells to insulin. Examples are pioglitazone (Actos) and rosiglitazone (Avandia).

tight glucose control—Achieving near normal levels of blood glucose by monitoring blood glucose several times a day and adjusting insulin doses accordingly. Aimed at preventing or slowing the progression of long-term complications of diabetes. Also called intensive glucose control.

type 1 diabetes—An autoimmune disease that destroys the ability of pancreatic beta cells to make insulin. Occurs most commonly in children and young adults. Daily insulin injections are necessary to stay alive.

type 2 diabetes—The most common type of diabetes; accounts for about 95% of all cases in the United States. Develops when the pancreas cannot make enough insulin to overcome the body's resistance to insulin action. Occurs most often in overweight or obese people over the age of 40, but its occurrence in overweight children is on the rise.

vitreous humor—A thick, gel-like substance that fills the back of the eyeball behind the lens.

HEALTH INFORMATION ORGANIZATIONS AND SUPPORT GROUPS

American Association of Diabetes Educators
100 West Monroe St., Suite 400
Chicago, IL 60603-1901
☎ 312-424-2426
www.aadenet.org
Organization of health professionals educating people on diabetes management. Provides books, programs, and referrals to local diabetes educators.

American Diabetes Association
Customer Service
1701 North Beauregard St.
Alexandria, VA 22311
☎ 800-342-2383
www.diabetes.org
National organization that funds research, provides information and publications, and offers referrals to support groups and education classes. Look in the white pages for your local chapter.

American Dietetic Association
216 W. Jackson Blvd.
Chicago, IL 60606-6995
☎ 800-366-1655/312-899-0040
www.eatright.org
Provides nutrition and weight control information, direct access to a registered dietitian, recorded nutrition messages, and referrals to local dietitians.

Joslin Diabetes Center
One Joslin Place
Boston, MA 02215
☎ 617-732-2400
www.joslin.harvard.edu
Part of the Harvard Medical School, the center is dedicated to treating diabetes. Has a research center; call the phone number for publications.

National Diabetes Information Clearinghouse
One Information Way
Bethesda, MD 20892-3560
☎ 800-860-8747
301-654-3327
www.niddk.nih.gov/health/diabetes/ndic.htm
Collects and disseminates information on diabetes. Responds to requests for information and provides publications.

National Institute of Diabetes and Digestive and Kidney Diseases
Office of Communications and Public Liaison
Building 31, Rm. 9A04
31 Center Drive, MSC 2560
Bethesda, MD 20892
www.niddk.nih.gov
Conducts and supports research on diabetes, as well as kidney, metabolic, and endocrine diseases.

National Kidney Foundation
30 East 33rd St., Suite 1100
New York, NY 10016
☎ 800-622-9010
212-889-2210
www.kidney.org
Health organization working for the prevention, treatment, and cure of kidney disease. Provides information and education on diabetes and kidney disease, as well as organ donation.

LEADING HOSPITALS FOR ENDOCRINOLOGY

U.S. News & World Report and the National Opinion Research Center, a social-science research group at the University of Chicago, recently conducted their 12th annual nationwide survey of 2,550 physicians in 17 medical specialties. The doctors nominated up to five hospitals they consider best from among 6,116 U.S. hospitals. This is the current list of the 10 best endocrinology hospitals, as determined by the doctors' recommendations from 1999, 2000, and 2001; federal data on death rates; and factual data regarding quality indicators, such as the ratio of registered nurses to patients and the use of advanced technology. Since the results reflect the doctors' opinions, however, they are, to some degree, subjective. Any institution listed is considered a leading center, and the rankings do not imply that other hospitals cannot or do not deliver excellent care.

1. **Mayo Clinic**
   Rochester, Minnesota
   www.mayo.edu/mcr/
   ☎ 507-284-2511
2. **Massachusetts General Hospital**
   Boston, Massachusetts
   www.mgh.harvard.edu
   ☎ 617-726-2000
3. **Johns Hopkins Hospital**
   Baltimore, Maryland
   www.hopkinsmedicine.org
   ☎ 410-955-5464/800-507-9952
4. **Brigham and Women's Hospital**
   Boston, Massachusetts
   www.brighamandwomens.org
   ☎ 617-732-5500
5. **Beth Israel Deaconess Medical Center**
   Boston, Massachusetts
   www.bidmc.harvard.edu
   ☎ 617-667-7000
6. **University of Virginia Health Sciences Center**
   Charlottesville, Virginia
   www.med.virginia.edu
   ☎ 804-924-3627/800-251-3627
7. **University of California, San Francisco Medical Center**
   San Francisco, California
   www.ucsfhealth.org
   ☎ 415-476-1000
8. **Barnes-Jewish Hospital**
   St. Louis, Missouri
   www.bjc.org
   ☎ 314-747-3000
9. **Cleveland Clinic**
   Cleveland, Ohio
   www.clevelandclinic.org
   ☎ 216-444-2200/800-223-2273
10. **University of Michigan Medical Center**
    Ann Arbor, Michigan
    www.med.umich.edu
    ☎ 734-936-4000

DIABETES AND MORTALITY IN WOMEN

Women are generally at lower risk for dying of coronary heart disease (CHD) than men. Women with diabetes, however, are an exception. Indeed, women with diabetes are just as likely to die of CHD-related causes as their male counterparts. Why diabetes boosts CHD risk is unclear. One possible explanation is that people with diabetes more often have blood lipid abnormalities, especially high triglycerides and low levels of high density lipoprotein (HDL, or "good," cholesterol), which increase the risk of CHD.

While there is plenty of evidence of a relationship between diabetes and an increased risk of heart disease, little research has been devoted to the impact diabetes has on the cause of death in women with the disease. The following study, reprinted from the American Medical Association's *Archives of Internal Medicine,* was aimed at filling this void.

Using data from the well-known Nurses' Health Study, researchers tracked 121,046 women for 20 years to determine how diabetes, as well as a prior history of CHD, affected mortality rates. The results were striking but not surprising. Women with both diabetes and CHD were nearly seven times more likely to die of any cause (not just heart-related causes) than those with neither condition. More dramatically, women with diabetes and CHD were 20 times more likely to die of cardiovascular causes (including stroke) and 25 times more likely to die of CHD than those with neither condition. The risk of dying of CHD increased proportionally with the number of years a woman had diabetes.

Women with preexisting CHD but no diabetes were somewhat—but not exceedingly—more likely to die of heart-related causes than those with diabetes but no CHD. This finding suggests that diabetes alone raises the risk of CHD-related death almost as much as having CHD alone. Furthermore, mortality from all causes was higher in women with diabetes alone than in those with CHD alone.

The take-home message from this study is that diabetes raises the risk of dying at an earlier age from any cause, but especially cardiovascular causes. The implication is that women with diabetes—especially those with a history of CHD—should be treated aggressively to reduce cardiovascular risk factors, such as high cholesterol, high blood pressure, cigarette smoking, and obesity. The large number of participants and the long, 20-year follow-up period make this study all the more reliable in its findings and authoritative in its conclusions.

The Impact of Diabetes Mellitus on Mortality From All Causes and Coronary Heart Disease in Women

20 Years of Follow-up

Frank B. Hu, MD; Meir J. Stampfer, MD; Caren G. Solomon, MD; Simin Liu, MD; Walter C. Willett, MD; Frank E. Speizer, MD; David M. Nathan, MD; JoAnn E. Manson, MD

Background: Few data are available on the long-term impact of type 2 diabetes mellitus on total mortality and fatal coronary heart disease (CHD) in women.

Methods: We examined prospectively the impact of type 2 diabetes and history of prior CHD on mortality from all causes and CHD among 121 046 women aged 30 to 55 years with type 2 diabetes in the Nurses' Health Study who were followed up for 20 years from 1976 to 1996.

Results: During 20 years of follow-up, we documented 8464 deaths from all causes, including 1239 fatal CHD events. Compared with women with no diabetes or CHD at baseline, age-adjusted relative risks (RRs) of overall mortality were 3.39 (95% confidence interval [CI], 3.08-3.73) for women with a history of diabetes and no CHD at baseline, 3.00 (95% CI, 2.50-3.60) for women with a history of CHD and no diabetes at baseline, and 6.84 (95% CI, 4.71-9.95) for women with both conditions at baseline. The corresponding age-adjusted RRs of fatal CHD across these 4 groups were 1.0, 8.70, 10.6, and 25.8, respectively. Multivariate adjustment for body mass index and other coronary risk factors only modestly attenuated the RRs. Compared with nondiabetic persons, the multivariate RRs of fatal CHD across categories of diabetes duration (≤5, 6-10, 11-15, 16-25, >25 years) were 2.75, 3.63, 5.51, 6.38, and 11.9 ($P<.001$ for trend), respectively. The combination of prior CHD and a long duration of clinical diabetes (ie, >15 years) was associated with a 30-fold (95% CI, 20.7-43.5) increased risk of fatal CHD.

Conclusions: Our data indicate that among women, history of diabetes is associated with dramatically increased risks of death from all causes and fatal CHD. The combination of diabetes and prior CHD identifies particularly high-risk women.

Arch Intern Med. 2001;161:1717-1723

TYPE 2 DIABETES mellitus is a well-established risk factor for coronary heart disease (CHD).[1] Diabetic women are at particularly high risk of CHD[2]; diabetes eliminates the usual female advantage for coronary disease mortality. Women with type 2 diabetes, compared with age-matched nondiabetic women, have a 5- to 7-fold higher rate of CHD death, with an event rate similar to that observed in men with type 2 diabetes.[3] Two recent analyses[4,5] have suggested that the magnitude of diabetes-related CHD mortality rivals the excess risk conferred by prior CHD. This finding challenges the National Cholesterol Education Program, which recommends more aggressive lipid-lowering therapy for people with prior CHD than for those with diabetes.[6] However, these studies were relatively small and did not consider duration of diabetes. Also, the results for diabetic men and women were combined, although it is known that diabetes confers a particularly high risk of CHD in women.[2]

The present study, with 20 years of follow-up, examines the impact of type 2 diabetes on mortality from all causes and from CHD among women in the Nurses' Health Study. In particular, we compared the risk of fatal CHD and total mortality among diabetic women without clinical CHD with that of women diagnosed as having CHD but not diabetes. We also examined the impact of duration of clinical diabetes on CHD risk.

RESULTS

During 20 years of follow-up from 1976 to 1996 (2 341 338 person-years), we documented 8464 deaths from all causes, including 1239 cases of fatal CHD. A total of 1892 deaths were ascribed to cardiovascular disease and 6572 were attributed to other causes (mainly cancer). **Table 1** presents characteristics of the participants in the middle year (1986) of the follow-up.

From the Departments of Nutrition (Drs Hu, Stampfer, and Willett) and Epidemiology (Drs Stampfer, Willett, and Manson), Harvard School of Public Health, Channing Laboratory (Drs Stampfer, Willett, Speizer, and Manson) and Divisions of Women's Health (Dr Solomon) and Preventive Medicine (Drs Liu and Manson), Department of Medicine, Brigham and Women's Hospital, and Diabetes Center (Dr Nathan), Massachusetts General Hospital, Harvard Medical School, Boston.

PARTICIPANTS AND METHODS

STUDY POPULATION

The Nurses' Health Study cohort was established in 1976 when 121 700 female registered nurses, aged 30 to 55 years and residing in 11 large states, completed a mailed questionnaire about their medical history and lifestyle. Every 2 years, follow-up questionnaires have been sent to update information on potential risk factors and to identify newly diagnosed cases of CHD and other illness. After excluding the relatively few women (n=343) whose diabetes was diagnosed at 30 years or younger (since they were most likely to have type 1 diabetes mellitus) and those with missing data on date of diagnosis of diabetes, the final population for analyses included 121 046 women.

ASSESSMENT OF HISTORY OF CHD

At baseline and every 2 years during follow-up, we asked the women to report whether they had angina pectoris, coronary bypass surgery or angioplasty, and/or myocardial infarction (MI). In this study, only report of a prior MI was considered as history of CHD. In 1976, 394 women reported a history of MI. During the follow-up from 1976 to 1994, 2473 women reported newly diagnosed MI. The confirmation of self-reported MI through medical record review according to strict diagnostic criteria was approximately 68% before 1984.[7] This increased to 82% between 1990 and 1996 (unpublished data). Most of the nonconfirmed cases had coronary disease but did not meet the criteria for MI.

CONFIRMATION OF DIABETES MELLITUS

In 1976, 1715 women reported physician-diagnosed diabetes (limited to diagnosis at age >30 years). During the follow-up periods, 6046 women reported newly diagnosed diabetes mellitus. A supplementary questionnaire regarding symptoms, diagnostic tests, and hypoglycemic therapy was mailed to women who indicated on any biennial questionnaire that they had been diagnosed as having diabetes. A case of diabetes was considered confirmed if at least 1 of the following was reported on the supplementary questionnaire: (1) 1 or more classic symptoms (excessive thirst, polyuria, weight loss, hunger, pruritus) plus fasting plasma glucose level of at least 140 mg/dL (7.8 mmol/L) or random plasma glucose level of at least 200 mg/dL (11.1 mmol/L); (2) at least 2 elevated plasma glucose concentrations on different occasions (fasting glucose level of at least 140 mg/dL or random plasma glucose level of at least 200 mg/dL and/or a concentration at least 200 mg/dL after 2 hours or more on oral glucose tolerance testing) in the absence of symptoms; or (3) treatment with hypoglycemic medication (insulin or oral hypoglycemic agent). The validity of this questionnaire has been verified in a subsample of this study population.[8] Among a random sample of 84 women classified by the questionnaire as having type 2 diabetes, 71 gave permission for their medical records to be reviewed and records were available for 62. An endocrinologist (J.E.M.), blinded to the information reported on the supplementary questionnaire, reviewed the records according to National Diabetes Data Group (NDDG) criteria.[9] The diagnosis of type 2 diabetes was confirmed in 61 (98%) of 62 women. Our primary analyses were based on self-reported diabetes. A secondary set of analyses was conducted that included only women with "definite" type 2 diabetes by the NDDG criteria. We used the NDDG diagnostic criteria because the analytic cohort preceded the American Diabetes Association's diagnostic guidelines published in 1997.[10]

ASCERTAINMENT OF END POINTS

The primary end points included deaths from all causes and fatal CHD that occurred after the return of the 1976

Women who had both diabetes and CHD were more likely to have hypertension and high cholesterol levels and less likely to use postmenopausal hormone therapy and vitamin E supplements. Women with a history of CHD, regardless of their diabetes status, were older and more likely to have a family history of CHD. On the other hand, women with a history of diabetes, regardless of CHD status, were heavier and drank less alcohol. Women with both diabetes and CHD were more likely to be treated with insulin than those with diabetes alone. Dietary intakes of fiber, fat, and cholesterol did not differ appreciably across the groups.

ANALYSES ACCORDING TO HISTORY OF DIABETES AND CHD AT BASELINE (1976)

At baseline in 1976, 1437 women reported diagnoses of diabetes (all these women were older than 30 years at diagnosis) and 394 reported diagnoses of MI. **Table 2** shows RRs of death from all causes, all cardiovascular disease, and fatal CHD according to diabetes and CHD status at baseline. The age-adjusted RR of all-cause mortality was approximately 7 times higher for women who had both diabetes and CHD compared with those with neither condition. The age-adjusted RR of death was 3.39 for women with a history of diabetes and no CHD compared with 3.00 for women with a history of CHD and no diabetes. Multivariate adjustment for smoking, body mass index, and other covariates somewhat attenuated these RRs. The multivariate-adjusted RRs of fatal CHD were similar for women with prior CHD (RR, 8.15; 95% confidence interval [CI], 6.25-10.6) and those with diabetes alone (RR, 7.48; 95% CI, 6.30-8.89). Women with both conditions were approximately 18 times more likely to die of CHD than those with neither conditions at baseline (multivariate RR, 17.6; 95% CI, 10.5-29.4).

ANALYSES ACCORDING TO UPDATED STATUS OF DIABETES AND CHD

During the follow-up periods, an additional 6046 women reported newly diagnosed diabetes (all these women were older than 30 years at diagnosis), and 2473 women reported newly diagnosed CHD. **Table 3** shows RRs of all-cause mortality, fatal CHD, and cardiovascular death according to diabetes and CHD diagnoses at baseline and during follow-up (updated every 2 years). Compared with women with neither diabetes nor CHD, multivariate RRs of all-cause mortality were 2.44 for women with diabe-

questionnaire but before June 1, 1996. Deaths were reported by next of kin and the postal system or ascertained through the National Death Index. We estimate that follow-up for the deaths was more than 98% complete.[11] We obtained copies of death certificates and medical records and determined causes of death (classified according to the categories of the *International Classification of Diseases, Ninth Revision* [*ICD-9*]).

Fatal CHD was confirmed by hospital records or autopsy or if CHD was listed as the cause of death on the death certificate and evidence of previous CHD was available. Probable fatal CHD cases were designated where CHD was the underlying cause on the death certificate, but no records were available. These cases constituted 14.7% of fatal CHD cases. We also included sudden deaths (12.3% of fatal CHD). Deaths owing to all cardiovascular disease included *ICD-9* codes 390 through 459 and 795.

STATISTICAL ANALYSIS

We conducted 2 sets of analyses, one comparing deaths from all causes and fatal CHD according to reported diabetes and CHD diagnoses at baseline (1976) and the other according to reported diagnoses either at baseline or during follow-up (updated every 2 years). Person-time for each participant was calculated from the date of return of the 1976 questionnaires to the date of confirmed fatal CHD, death from other causes, or June 1, 1996, whichever came first.

We calculated rates of fatal CHD for women with prior diabetes, CHD, or both by dividing the number of incident cases by the number of person-years of follow-up. The relative risk (RR) was computed as the rate among women with prior diabetes, CHD, or both divided by the rate among women with neither condition, with adjustment for 5-year age categories. For the analysis of overall mortality, person-time was calculated from the date of the 1976 questionnaire to the date of death from any cause or June 1, 1996. Duration of clinical diabetes was calculated as years since first diagnosis of diabetes and the variable was divided into 5 categories (≤5, 6-10, 11-15, 16-25, >25 years). We collapsed the last 2 categories in the analysis of duration of diabetes stratified by prior CHD. Test for trend was conducted by treating the original duration variable as a continuous variable.

We used pooled logistic regression to adjust estimated incidence rate ratios simultaneously for potential confounding variables. In this approach, independent 2-year blocks of person-time of follow-up are pooled for regression analysis, and the dependence of the incidence rates on time is modeled nonparametrically with indicator variables. D'Agostino et al[12] have showed that the pooled logistic model is asymptotically equivalent to the Cox regression when the time intervals are short and the probability of outcome in the intervals is low (both assumptions are satisfied by our data); examples comparing the 2 methods were given by Cupples et al.[13] Our covariates included age (5-year categories); body mass index, a measure of weight in kilograms divided by the square of height in meters (<21, 21-22.9, 23-24.9, 25-28.9, 29-31.9, ≥32); cigarette smoking (never, past, and current smoking of 1 to 14, 15 to 24, and ≥25 cigarettes per day); menopausal status (premenopausal, postmenopausal without hormone replacement, postmenopausal with past hormone replacement, postmenopausal with current hormone replacement); and parental history of MI before the age of 60 years. We did not adjust for history of hypertension or hypercholesterolemia because they are considered intermediate variables in the biological pathway. Secondary analysis further adjusting for these variables did not materially change the RRs for total mortality but somewhat attenuated the RRs for fatal CHD. All covariates except parental history of MI were updated every 2 years. Alcohol use and physical activity were first assessed in 1980. Because further analyses adjusting for these 2 variables did not alter the results, we did not include them in the final model. As preplanned, we conducted stratified analyses according to age group, history of hypertension, high cholesterol levels, and parental history of MI.

tes alone, 2.58 for women with CHD alone, and 5.82 for women with both conditions. Compared with women with neither conditions, women with both diabetes and prior CHD were 20 times more likely to die from any cardiovascular disease and 25 times more likely to die from CHD. In contrast to results from Table 2, the RRs of cardiovascular death and fatal CHD were substantially greater for women with CHD alone than those with diabetes alone. The multivariate RRs of fatal CHD were 10.7 (95% CI, 9.03-12.6) for women with CHD alone compared with 5.65 (95% CI, 4.83-6.60) for women with diabetes alone. Restriction of the analyses to only patients with diabetes confirmed by the supplementary questionnaires did not appreciably alter the results. (The age-adjusted RRs of fatal CHD were 12.0 for women with CHD alone and 6.19 for women with diabetes alone.)

In subgroup analyses, the excess risk of fatal CHD associated with diabetes alone, prior CHD alone, or both was significant in all subgroups stratified by age group, history of hypertension, history of high cholesterol levels, or parental history of MI (**Table 4**). Compared with younger women (<55 years) with neither condition, the RR of fatal CHD for older women (≥65 years) with both diabetes and existing CHD was 159.5 (95% CI, 111.1-229.1). As expected, history of hypertension and parental history of MI augmented the elevated RRs associated with diabetes alone or prior CHD. Interestingly, for women who had diabetes or CHD, high cholesterol levels did not appear to further increase the risk of fatal CHD. One possible explanation is that cholesterol-lowering treatment may have already reduced the risk among those patients.

THE IMPACT OF DURATION OF CLINICAL DIABETES

The risk of CHD mortality increased monotonically with increased duration of clinical diabetes (**Figure 1**). Compared with nondiabetic women, the RRs of fatal CHD across categories of duration of diabetes (≤5, 6-10, 11-15, 16-25, >25 years) were 2.75, 3.63, 5.51, 6.38, and 11.9 ($P<.001$ for trend). In the same multivariate model, the RR of fatal CHD for women with vs without prior CHD was 5.49. The increased risk of fatal CHD with longer duration of diabetes, especially among those with diabetes for 15 years or more, was persistent in women with or without prior CHD (**Figure 2**). Women with prior CHD alone had a RR of 8.61 (95% CI, 7.08-10.5), which was similar to that among women with diabetes for more

Table 1. Distribution of Potential Coronary Risk Factors According to History of Diabetes and Coronary Heart Disease (CHD) in 1986*

Risk Factor	No Diabetes and No CHD	Diabetes and No CHD	CHD and No Diabetes	Diabetes and CHD
No. of women	109 231	3705	1302	234
Current smokers, %	23.6	21.0	27.1	19.4
History of hypertension, %	23.1	55.9	47.7	77.4
History of hypercholesterolemia, %	11.2	28.2	32.9	55.0
Parental MI before 60 y, %	20.0	24.1	31.1	29.4
Insulin treatment, %	. . .	25.8	. . .	33.9
Oral hypoglycemic medications, %	. . .	32.4	. . .	27.5
Current postmenopausal hormone use among postmenopausal women, %	19.0	17.1	19.4	14.3
Multivitamin use, %	42.5	41.9	38.4	35.8
Vitamin E supplement use, %	16.2	15.0	12.6	9.2
Age, mean, y	59.9	63.1	65.1	65.8
Alcohol use, mean, g/d	6.3	3.0	6.0	1.5
BMI, mean	25.2	29.8	26.7	30.4
Hours of moderate or vigorous exercise per week, mean	3.1	2.8	2.8	2.7
Dietary fiber intake, mean, g/d	19.1	19.9	20.0	20.1
Saturated fat intake, mean, % energy	11.7	12.0	11.1	11.2
Polyunsaturated fat intake, mean, % energy	6.2	6.2	5.9	5.9
Trans fat intake, mean, % energy	1.7	1.7	1.5	1.6
Dietary cholesterol intake, mean, mg/1000 kcal	150	168	148	164

*The year 1986 was used in this analysis to represent the overall follow-up of the cohort (1976-1996). Percentages and means for variables other than age are standardized according to the age distribution of the overall study group. MI indicates myocardial infarction; BMI, body mass index (a measure of weight in kilograms divided by the square of height in meters).

Reported in the supplementary questionnaire or 1998 main questionnaire.

Table 2. Relative Risks of Death From All Causes, CHD, and All Cardiovascular Disease According to History of Diabetes and Prior CHD at Baseline in 1976: The Nurses' Health Study, 1976-1996*

Type of Death	No Diabetes and No CHD	Diabetes and No CHD	CHD and No Diabetes	Diabetes and CHD
Deaths from all causes				
No. of cases	7853	458	123	30
Person-years	2 300 753	31 641	7997	948
RR (95% CI)				
Age adjusted	1.0	3.39 (3.08-3.73)	3.00 (2.50-3.60)	6.84 (4.71-9.95)
Multivariate	1.0	3.12 (2.83-3.44)	2.55 (2.12-3.07)	5.08 (3.47-7.43)
All cardiovascular deaths				
No. of cases	1582	216	75	19
RR (95% CI)				
Age adjusted	1.0	7.51 (6.50-8.67)	8.40 (6.63-10.6)	19.9 (12.5-31.8)
Multivariate	1.0	6.59 (5.69-7.63)	6.58 (5.19-8.36)	13.6 (8.45-21.8)
Fatal CHD				
No. of cases	1001	161	61	16
RR (95% CI)				
Age adjusted	1.0	8.70 (7.35-10.3)	10.6 (8.14-13.8)	25.8 (15.6-42.9)
Multivariate	1.0	7.48 (6.30-8.89)	8.15 (6.25-10.6)	17.6 (10.5-29.4)

*CHD indicates coronary heart disease; RR, relative risk; and CI, confidence interval.

Models include the following: age (5-year category); time (10 periods); body mass index, a measure of weight in kilograms divided by the square of height in meters (<21, 21-22.9, 23-24.9, 25-28.9, 29-31.9, ≥32); cigarette smoking (never, past, and current smoking of 1 to 14, 15 to 24, and ≥25 cigarettes per day); menopausal status (premenopausal, postmenopausal without hormone replacement, postmenopausal with past hormone replacement, postmenopausal with current hormone replacement); and parental history of myocardial infarction before 60 years of age.

Deaths due to all cardiovascular disease included *International Classification of Diseases, Ninth Edition* codes 390 through 459 and 795.

than 15 years (RR, 8.66; 95% CI, 6.87-10.9). A combination of CHD and a long duration of diabetes (ie, >15 years) identifies a particularly high-risk group for fatal CHD (RR, 30.0; 95% CI, 20.7-43.5).

In contrast to the monotonic increased risk of fatal CHD with longer duration of diabetes, the risk of fatal CHD increased dramatically in the first several years after onset of an MI and then remained relatively stable; compared with women without a prior MI, the multivariate RRs of fatal CHD across categories of number of years after first MI (≤5, 6-10, 11-20, >20 years) were 4.70, 6.05, 6.12, and 6.74, respectively.

COMMENT

In this large prospective cohort of women, type 2 diabetes mellitus was associated with dramatically increased mortality from all causes and fatal CHD among women.

Table 3. Relative Risks of Death From All Causes, CHD, and All Cardiovascular Disease According to the Status of Diabetes and CHD at Baseline and During Follow-up: The Nurses' Health Study, 1976-1996*

Type of Death	No Diabetes and No CHD	Diabetes and No CHD	CHD and No Diabetes	Diabetes and CHD
Deaths from all causes				
No. of cases	6939	878	408	239
Person-years	2 231 377	76 356	27 169	6435
RR (95% CI)				
Age adjusted	1.0	2.47 (2.30-2.65)	2.75 (2.48-3.04)	6.12 (5.34-7.00)
Multivariate	1.0	2.44 (2.27-2.63)	2.58 (2.33-2.87)	5.82 (5.07-6.69)
All cardiovascular deaths				
No. of cases	1188	325	221	158
RR (95% CI)				
Age adjusted	1.0	5.11 (4.51-5.80)	8.23 (7.10-9.54)	22.1 (18.6-26.3)
Multivariate	1.0	4.86 (4.27-5.52)	7.46 (6.43-8.66)	20.1 (16.8-24.1)
Fatal CHD				
No. of cases	697	231	189	122
RR (95% CI)				
Age adjusted	1.0	6.19 (5.32-7.20)	12.0 (10.2-14.2)	29.0 (23.7-35.5)
Multivariate	1.0	5.65 (4.83-6.60)	10.7 (9.03-12.6)	25.3 (20.6-31.1)

*CHD indicates coronary heart disease; RR, relative risk; and CI, confidence interval. The diagnoses of diabetes and CHD were updated every 2 years.
Models include the following: age (5-year category); time (10 periods); body mass index (5 categories); cigarette smoking (never, past, and current smoking of 1 to 14, 15 to 24, and ≥25 cigarettes per day); menopausal status (premenopausal, postmenopausal without hormone replacement, postmenopausal with past hormone replacement, postmenopausal with current hormone replacement); and parental history of myocardial infarction before 60 years of age.

Table 4. Multivariate Relative Risks (95% Confidence Intervals) of CHD Death According to the Status of Diabetes and CHD at Baseline and During Follow-up: Subgroup Analysis*

	No Diabetes and No CHD	Diabetes and No CHD	CHD and No Diabetes	Diabetes and CHD
Age groups, y				
<55 (n = 250)	1.0 (Referent)	9.19 (6.39-13.2)	29.2 (19.7-43.3)	87.0 (51.3-147.4)
55-64 (n = 591)	3.92 (3.16-4.88)	21.5 (16.4-28.3)	44.4 (33.3-58.9)	105.5 (75.3-148.0)
≥65 (n = 398)	8.83 (6.81-11.4)	42.7 (31.4-58.1)	66.3 (47.8-92.0)	159.5 (111.1-229.1)
History of hypertension				
No (n = 419)	1.0 (Referent)	5.51 (3.97-7.63)	15.3 (11.6-20.2)	51.5 (32.1-82.6)
Yes (n = 820)	3.45 (2.95-4.03)	13.3 (10.9-16.2)	23.0 (18.5-28.7)	48.8 (38.2-62.2)
History of high cholesterol levels				
No (n = 732)	1.0 (Referent)	5.68 (4.61-6.99)	11.8 (9.30-14.9)	32.0 (22.7-45.3)
Yes (n = 507)	1.42 (1.19-1.69)	7.09 (5.71-8.81)	12.1 (9.65-15.1)	27.3 (21.2-35.1)
Parental history of myocardial infarction				
No (n = 927)	1.0 (Referent)	5.86 (4.92-6.98)	11.1 (9.05-13.5)	26.5 (20.7-33.8)
Yes (n = 312)	1.65 (1.38-1.97)	8.22 (6.14-11.0)	16.1 (12.3-21.0)	37.4 (26.7-52.3)

*Adjusted for the same variables as in Table 3; n indicates the number of coronary heart disease (CHD) deaths. The total number of fatal CHD cases does not add to 1239 because of missing data on menopausal status.
Age was entered as a continuous variable in the stratified analyses.

We observed a strong monotonic relationship between duration of clinical diabetes and CHD mortality, independent of history of CHD. The combination of a long duration of diabetes and preexisting CHD identifies a particularly high-risk group.

Several previous studies have compared the magnitude of CHD risk associated with history of diabetes or prior CHD. Haffner et al[4] followed up 2432 Finnish men and women aged 45 to 64 years for 7 years and found that the risk of fatal CHD was as high among diabetic patients without prior CHD as it was among nondiabetic patients who had experienced prior CHD. Because the study involved only 69 nondiabetic patients with prior CHD, the power of the study to detect differences between the 2 groups was limited. Also, the small sample size did not allow separate analyses by sex or stratification by duration of diabetes. In a 5-year follow-up of 91 285 US male physicians aged 40 to 84 years, Lotufo et al[14] found that for all-cause mortality, the magnitude of excess risk conferred by diabetes was similar to that conferred by prior CHD. For fatal CHD, however, prior CHD was a more powerful predictor (age-adjusted RR was 3.3 for diabetic men without prior CHD vs 5.6 for nondiabetic men with prior CHD). The discrepancy of the results between the 2 studies may be due to different age distribution and sex composition of the 2 populations. The duration of diabetes may also be different in the 2 studies; the average duration of diabetes was 8 years in the Finnish study, whereas the duration of diabetes was not ascertained in the Physicians' Health Study. Re-

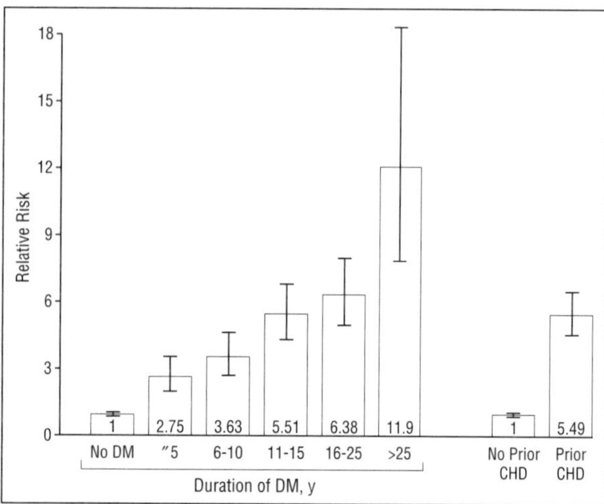

Figure 1. Multivariate relative risks and 95% confidence intervals of fatal coronary heart disease (CHD) associated with duration of diabetes mellitus (DM) and a prior history of CHD. Adjusted for the same covariates as in Table 2.

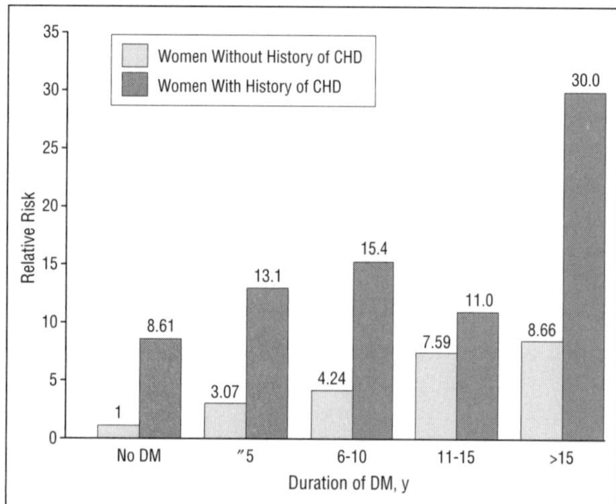

Figure 2. Multivariate relative risks of fatal coronary heart disease (CHD) according to duration of diabetes mellitus (DM) stratified by a prior history of CHD. Adjusted for the same covariates as in Table 2.

cently, Malmberg and colleagues[5] reported that in a 2-year study diabetic patients (duration of diabetes was not specified) without prior cardiovascular disease had rates of coronary morbidity and mortality similar to those for nondiabetic patients with previous vascular disease.

In our baseline analyses (Table 2), the excess risk of cardiovascular death and fatal CHD conferred by diabetes alone was similar to that conferred by prior CHD. However, in the updated analyses (Table 3), the excess risk of fatal CHD associated with preexisting CHD was substantially greater than that conferred by diabetes without clinical CHD. Obviously, in the baseline analyses, only women who had a long duration of diabetes (≥20 years) were included in the diabetic group, whereas in the updated analyses, both new and long-standing cases of diabetes were included. Our findings highlight the importance of considering duration of diabetes when comparing the magnitude of excess risk of fatal CHD conferred by diabetes alone and prior CHD.

Diabetes has more deleterious effects on women than on men; it eliminates the usual female advantage for coronary disease mortality. In the Rancho Bernardo Study,[15] diabetic women had CHD mortality rates similar to both nondiabetic and diabetic men, whereas nondiabetic women had substantially lower risk. The reason for the accelerated atherogenesis among diabetic women is not completely understood, but it is at least in part related to more severe lipid and lipoprotein abnormalities, particularly elevated levels of triglycerides and reduced levels of high-density lipoprotein, among diabetic women.[16,17] A recent study[3] suggests greater impairment of endothelial function associated with type 2 diabetes in women than in men. In addition, the magnitude of increased risk of reinfarction and fatality rate following an acute MI among diabetic patients compared with nondiabetic patients was greater in women than in men.[18]

Our data support current guidelines that recommend aggressive management of cardiovascular risk factors in diabetic patients, including hypertension, dyslipidemia, and lifestyle factors (smoking, obesity, and diet).[19] The United Kingdom Prospective Diabetes Study showed that tight control of blood pressure substantially decreased the risk of diabetes-related deaths and the progression of microvascular complications,[20] providing support for tighter control of blood pressure for diabetic individuals than usually is recommended for nondiabetic individuals with hypertension.

A recent American Diabetes Association guideline[21] recommends the same cholesterol-lowering goal for people with diabetes and no clinical CHD as for patients with preexisting CHD (ie, a low-density lipoprotein cholesterol level <100 mg/dL [<2.59 mmol/L]). Two statin trials[22,23] among patients with existing CHD showed similar significant reductions in CHD death in both patients with and without diabetes. A secondary analysis of the Scandinavian Simvastatin Survival Study showed that simvastatin therapy was associated with even greater reductions in risk of major CHD events and total mortality among diabetic patients than among nondiabetic patients.[24] The effects of tight glycemic control on cardiovascular complications are not yet settled, although intensive therapy that lowers blood glucose levels has been proved to reduce risk of microvascular complications in both patients with type 1[25] and type 2[26] diabetes.

Our study is one of few epidemiologic studies on diabetes-related cardiovascular risk among women. The large sample size and long duration of follow-up provide the opportunity to examine the impact of duration of clinical diabetes on risk of cardiovascular disease. The follow-up rate of this cohort was high during 20 years of follow-up (98% for death ascertainment). Thus, our study results are unlikely to be biased by losses to follow-up. In addition, we have collected detailed information on cardiovascular risk factors such as smoking, body mass index, menopausal status, and postmenopausal hormone use through repeated assessments.

Several limitations of the study should be considered. The data on diagnosed diabetes and CHD were based on self-reports by the nurses. This may have led to some misclassification. However, our previous studies[7,8] have found self-reporting of these medical conditions to be reliable. To avoid potential confounding by type 1 diabetes, we included only women reporting a diagnosis of diabetes at 30 years or older. Moreover, the analysis restricted to confirmed cases of type 2 diabetes by the supplementary questionnaire yielded similar results.

Because our "nondiabetic" cohort was not uniformly screened for glucose intolerance and the onset of diabetes can occur several years before clinical diagnosis,[27] the reported duration of diabetes in our study may have been underestimated. Also, some cases of diabetes may have been undiagnosed. This misclassification, however, would have inflated the cardiovascular risk in the nondiabetic population and led to underestimation of the RRs among our diabetic population. We believe that the proportion of undiagnosed diabetes is relatively small in our cohort compared with the general population because virtually all participants in our study have ready access to health care. For example, more than 98% of the women in our study visited a physician for a physical examination, breast examination, mammogram, or sigmoidoscopy or colonoscopy at least once between 1988 and 1990. Finally, the diagnostic criteria for type 2 diabetes were changed in 1997[10] such that lower fasting glucose levels (≥126 mg/dL [≥6.99 mmol/L]) would now be considered diagnostic. We used the criteria proposed by the National Diabetes Data Group[9] because all our cases were diagnosed before June 1996. If the new criteria were used, some women in this study classified as nondiabetic would have been reclassified as having diabetes, and the cardiovascular risk in the reference (nondiabetic) population would have been even lower.

In conclusion, our data indicate that diabetes is associated with dramatically increased risk of total mortality and CHD death among women. The excess risk of fatal CHD for women who had clinical diabetes for more than 15 years was similar to that conferred by prior CHD. The combination of a long duration of diabetes and preexisting CHD identifies a particularly high-risk group.

Accepted for publication January 18, 2001.

This study was supported by research grants DK36798, HL24074, HL34594, and CA40356 from the National Institutes of Health, Bethesda, Md. Dr Hu's work is supported by an American Diabetes Association Research Award. Dr Solomon is supported by an American Heart Association Clinician Scientist Award.

We are indebted to the participants in the Nurses' Health Study for their continuing outstanding level of cooperation and to Al Wing, MBA, Gary Chase, Karen Corsano, MSL, Lisa Dunn, Barbara Egan, Lori Ward, Erin Boyd, and Jill Arnold for their unfailing help.

Corresponding author: Frank B. Hu, MD, Department of Nutrition, Harvard School of Public Health, 665 Huntington Ave, Boston, MA 02115 (e-mail: Frank.hu@channing.harvard.edu).

REFERENCES

1. Grundy SM, Benjamin IJ, Burke GL, et al. Diabetes and cardiovascular disease: a statement for healthcare professionals from the American Heart Association. *Circulation.* 1999;100:1134-1146.
2. Manson JE, Spelsberg A. Risk modification in the diabetic patient. In: Manson JE, Ridker PM, Gaziano JM, Hennekens CH, eds. *Prevention of Myocardial Infarction.* New York, NY: Oxford University Press; 1996:241-273.
3. Steinberg HO, Paradisi G, Cronin J, et al. Type II diabetes abrogates sex differences in endothelial function in premenopausal women. *Circulation.* 2000;101:2040-2046.
4. Haffner SM, Lehto S, Ronnemaa T, Pyorala K, Laakso M. Mortality from coronary heart disease in subjects with type 2 diabetes and in nondiabetic subjects with and without prior myocardial infarction. *N Engl J Med.* 1998;339:229-234.
5. Malmberg K, Yusuf S, Gerstein HC, et al. Impact of diabetes on long-term prognosis in patients with unstable angina and non±Q-wave myocardial infarction: results of the OASIS (Organization to Assess Strategies for Ischemic Syndromes) Registry. *Circulation.* 2000;102:1014-1019.
6. Expert Panel on Detection, Evaluation, and Treatment of High Blood Cholesterol in Adults. Summary of the second report of the National Cholesterol Education Program (NCEP) Expert Panel on Detection, Evaluation, and Treatment of High Blood Cholesterol in Adults (Adult Treatment Panel II). *JAMA.* 1993;209:3015-3023.
7. Colditz GA, Martin P, Stampfer MJ, et al. Validation of questionnaire information on risk factors and disease outcomes in a prospective cohort study of women. *Am J Epidemiol.* 1986;123:894-900.
8. Manson JE, Colditz GA, Stampfer MJ, et al. A prospective study of maturity-onset diabetes mellitus and risk of coronary heart disease and stroke in women. *Arch Intern Med.* 1991;151:1141-1147.
9. National Diabetes Data Group. Classification and diagnosis of diabetes mellitus and other categories of glucose intolerance. *Diabetes.* 1979;28:1039-1057.
10. Expert Committee on the Diagnosis and Classification of Diabetes Mellitus. Report of the Expert Committee on the Diagnosis and Classification of Diabetes Mellitus. *Diabetes Care.* 1997;20:1183-1194.
11. Stampfer MJ, Willett WC, Speizer FE, et al. Test of the National Death Index. *Am J Epidemiol.* 1984;119:837-839.
12. D'Agostino RB, Lee M-L, Belanger AJ, Cupples LA, Anderson K, Kannel WB. Relation of pooled logistic regression to time dependent Cox regression analysis: the Framingham Heart Study. *Stat Med.* 1990;9:1501-1515.
13. Cupples LA, D'Agostino RB, Anderson K, Kannel WB. Comparison of baseline and repeated measure covariate techniques in the Framingham Heart Study. *Stat Med.* 1988;7:205-222.
14. Lotufo PA, Gaziano JM, Chae CU, et al. Diabetes and all-cause and coronary heart disease mortality among US male physicians. *Arch Intern Med.* 2001;161:242-247.
15. Barrett-Connor E, Cohn BA, Wingard DL, Edelstein S. Why is diabetes a stronger risk factor for fatal ischemic heart disease in women than in men? the Rancho Bernardo Study. *JAMA.* 1991;265:627-631.
16. Walden CE, Knopp RH, Wahl PW. Sex differences in the effect of diabetes mellitus on lipoprotein triglyceride and cholesterol concentrations. *N Engl J Med.* 1984;311:953-959.
17. Siegel RD, Cupples A, Schaefer EJ, Wilson WF. Lipoproteins, apolipoproteins, and low-density lipoprotein size among diabetics in the Framingham Offspring Study. *Metabolism.* 1996;10:1267-1272.
18. Abott RD, Donahue RP, Kannel WB, Wilson PWF. The impact of diabetes on survival following myocardial infarction in men vs women: the Framingham Study. *JAMA.* 1988;23:3456-3460.
19. American Diabetes Association. Clinical practice recommendations 2000. *Diabetes Care.* 2000;23:S1-S116.
20. United Kingdom Prospective Diabetes Study Group. Tight blood pressure control and the risk of macrovascular and microvascular complications in type 2 diabetes: UKPDS 38. *BMJ.* 1998;317:703-720.
21. American Diabetes Association. Management of dyslipidemia in adults with diabetes. *Diabetes Care.* 2000;23(suppl 1):S57-S60.
22. Goldberg RB, Mellies MJ, Sacks FM, et al. Cardiovascular events and their reduction with pravastatin in diabetic and glucose-intolerant myocardial infarction survivors with average cholesterol levels: subgroup analyses in the Cholesterol And Recurrent Events (CARE) trial. *Circulation.* 1998;98:2513-2519.
23. The Long-term Intervention with Pravastatin in Ischemic Disease (LIPID) Study Group. Prevention of cardiovascular events and death with pravastatin in patients with coronary heart disease and a broad range of initial cholesterol levels. *N Engl J Med.* 1998;339:1349-1357.
24. Pyorala K, Pedersen TR, Kjekshus J, Faergeman O, Olsson AG, Thorgiersson G. Cholesterol lowering with simvastatin improves prognosis of diabetes with coronary heart disease. *Diabetes Care.* 1997;20:614-620.
25. The Diabetes Control and Complications Trial Research Group. The effect of intensive treatment of diabetes on the development and progression of long-term complications in insulin-dependent diabetes mellitus. *N Engl J Med.* 1993;329:977-986.
26. UK Prospective Diabetes Study Group. Effect of intensive blood-glucose control with metformin on complications in overweight patients with type 2 diabetes (UKPDS 34). *Lancet.* 1998;352:854-865.
27. Harris MI, Klein R, Welborn TA, Knuiman MW. Onset of NIDDM occurs at least 4-7 yr before clinical diagnosis. *Diabetes Care.* 1992;15:815-819.

NOTES

NOTES

NOTES

NOTES

NOTES

NOTES

NOTES

NOTES

The information contained in this White Paper is not intended as a substitute for the advice of a physician. Readers who suspect they may have specific medical problems should consult a physician about any suggestions made.

Please address inquiries on bulk subscriptions and permission to reproduce selections from this White Paper to Medletter Associates, Inc., 632 Broadway, 11th Floor, New York, NY 10012. The editors are interested in receiving your comments at the above address, but regret that they cannot answer letters of any sort personally.

ISBN 0-929661-16-8
Eighth Printing
Printed in the United States of America

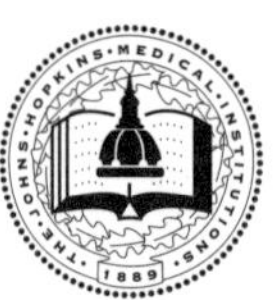

The Johns Hopkins White Papers are published yearly by Medletter Associates, Inc.

Rodney Friedman	Publisher
Devon Schuyler	Executive Editor
Catherine Richter	Senior Editor
Paul Candon	Senior Writer
Maureen O'Sullivan	Writer/Researcher
Kimberly Flynn	Writer/Researcher
Liz Curry	Editorial Associate
Marcie Lipper	Intern
Leslie Maltese-McGill	Copy Editor
Bonnie Slotnick	Copy Editor
Scott Hunt	Design Production Manager
Robert Duckwall	Medical Illustrator
Mark Desierto	Librarian
Barbara Maxwell O'Neill	Associate Publisher
Helen Mullen	Circulation Director
David Alexander	Circulation Manager
Jerry Loo	Product Manager
Allison Hordos	Promotions Coordinator
Joan Mullally	Head of Business Development

The 2002 White Papers

62B11A

Take Control of Your Medical Condition

Visit us online at www.HealthAfter50.com

YES, I've placed a check mark next to the White Paper(s) I'd like to receive for $24.95 each. Annual updates on each subject that I have chosen will be offered to me by announcement card. I need do nothing if I want the update to be sent to me automatically. If I do not want it, I will return the announcement card marked "cancel." I may cancel at any time. (Please add $2.95 for domestic, $4.95 for Canadian, and $15.00 for foreign orders to your total to cover shipping and handling.) (Florida residents add sales tax.)

✔ **Please put a check mark next to the White Paper(s) you wish to order.**

001024 ❑	Arthritis	$24.95	008029 ❑	Prostate Disorders	$24.95
003020 ❑	Coronary Heart Disease	$24.95	010025 ❑	Disgestive Disorders	$24.95
004028 ❑	Depression and Anxiety	$24.95	011023 ❑	Vision	$24.95
005025 ❑	Diabetes	$24.95	012021 ❑	Low Back Pain & Osteoporosis	$24.95
006023 ❑	Hypertension and Stroke	$24.95	015024 ❑	Memory	$24.95

METHOD OF PAYMENT: (U.S. funds only) ❑ VISA ❑ MasterCard ❑ Check Enclosed ❑ Bill me

Name

Address

City State Zip

Credit Card # Exp. Date

Signature Date

Money Back Guarantee: If for any reason, you are not satisfied after receipt of your publications, return your purchase within 30 days for a full refund.

Detach and mail this card back to The Johns Hopkins White Papers, P.O. Box 420083, Palm Coast, FL 32142

The 2002 White Papers

62B11A

Take Control of Your Medical Condition

Visit us online at www.HealthAfter50.com

YES, I've placed a check mark next to the White Paper(s) I'd like to receive for $24.95 each. Annual updates on each subject that I have chosen will be offered to me by announcement card. I need do nothing if I want the update to be sent to me automatically. If I do not want it, I will return the announcement card marked "cancel." I may cancel at any time. (Please add $2.95 for domestic, $4.95 for Canadian, and $15.00 for foreign orders to your total to cover shipping and handling.) (Florida residents add sales tax.)

✔ **Please put a check mark next to the White Paper(s) you wish to order.**

001024 ❑	Arthritis	$24.95	008029 ❑	Prostate Disorders	$24.95
003020 ❑	Coronary Heart Disease	$24.95	010025 ❑	Disgestive Disorders	$24.95
004028 ❑	Depression and Anxiety	$24.95	011023 ❑	Vision	$24.95
005025 ❑	Diabetes	$24.95	012021 ❑	Low Back Pain & Osteoporosis	$24.95
006023 ❑	Hypertension and Stroke	$24.95	015024 ❑	Memory	$24.95

METHOD OF PAYMENT: (U.S. funds only) ❑ VISA ❑ MasterCard ❑ Check Enclosed ❑ Bill me

Name

Address

City State Zip

Credit Card # Exp. Date

Signature Date

Money Back Guarantee: If for any reason, you are not satisfied after receipt of your publications, return your purchase within 30 days for a full refund.

Detach and mail this card back to The Johns Hopkins White Papers, P.O. Box 420083, Palm Coast, FL 32142

Johns
Hopkins
White Papers

Fold along this line and tape closed

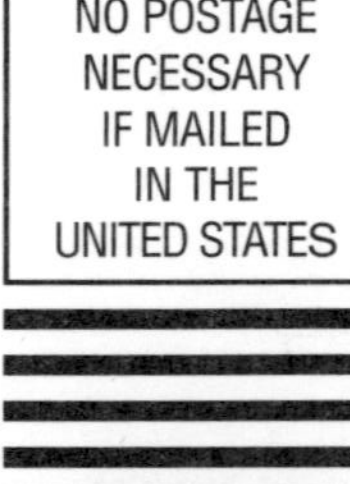

NO POSTAGE
NECESSARY
IF MAILED
IN THE
UNITED STATES

BUSINESS REPLY MAIL
FIRST-CLASS MAIL PERMIT NO. 86 FLAGLER BEACH FL

POSTAGE WILL BE PAID BY ADDRESSEE

THE JOHNS HOPKINS WHITE PAPERS
PO BOX 420083
PALM COAST FL 32142-9264

Johns
Hopkins
White Papers

Fold along this line and tape closed

NO POSTAGE
NECESSARY
IF MAILED
IN THE
UNITED STATES

BUSINESS REPLY MAIL
FIRST-CLASS MAIL PERMIT NO. 86 FLAGLER BEACH FL

POSTAGE WILL BE PAID BY ADDRESSEE

THE JOHNS HOPKINS WHITE PAPERS
PO BOX 420083
PALM COAST FL 32142-9264